Advance Praise for *A Field Manual for Palliative Care in Humanitarian Crises*

"This field guide is a rich and timely tool that embraces the holistic approach to addressing the palliative care needs of people in humanitarian crises. By positioning the guide as a trauma-informed response to humanitarian crises, the authors put an all-round and handy tool in our hands for a cause that is so often neglected yet so common on all continents. In addition, the guide is comprehensive and does not miss the needs of children as another key component. I highly recommend it to all involved in care in emergency and humanitarian situations."

—Emmanuel B.K. Luyirika, MBChB, BPA (Hons), MPA, MFamMed,
Executive Director, African Palliative Care Association,
Kampala, Uganda

"Much too often in any humanitarian crisis, the rescued are left to live a life that feels worse than death to them. Waldman and Glass show us how such lives could be made worth living, with a little planning, preparation, genuine concern, and care. A most essential guide to all involved in the management of humanitarian crisis and in palliative care."

—M.R. Rajagopal, MD,
Chairman, Pallium India,
Director, World Health Organization Collaborating Centre for Training and
Policy on Access to Pain Relief,
Thiruvananthapuram, India

"Not only is this book an incredibly useful resource and reference for providing high-quality palliative care in resource-limited settings, it shines light on the importance of incorporating a focus of relief of suffering when providing care in a time of crisis. This book can help guide everyone from community health workers to physicians to provide better care for their patients, and in highlighting what is possible, serves as an inspiration to bring this care to settings where it is needed most."

—Timothy Poore, MD,
Assistant Clinical Professor of Medicine,
Division of Palliative Medicine, University of California, San Francisco,
San Francisco, CA

"Waldman and Glass's *The Field Manual for Palliative Care in Humanitarian Crises* fills a critically important gap in the care of seriously ill patients of all ages facing extreme circumstances. The promotion of generalists' palliative care skills among the highly devoted healthcare responders will greatly enhance the care of those in need. As a pediatrician, I am especially impressed by the focus on the needs of children and attention to pediatric dosing throughout the manual. I commend the authors for this vital contribution."

—Joanne Wolfe, MD, MPH,
Director, Pediatric Palliative Care, Boston Children's Hospital,
Division Chief, Pediatric Palliative Care Service,
Department of Psychosocial Oncology and Palliative Care,
Dana-Farber Cancer Institute,
Boston, MA

"The uncomfortable necessity of a reference like this, that provides boots-on-the-ground recommendations for those providing healthcare in humanitarian crises, is only offset by the welcome, recent, global recognition that, the aggressive allevi-ation of suffering for those patients that may or may not long survive is as impor-tant as saving lives. This guide enables groups to anticipate disasters and create readiness plans and provides a framework, after a disaster may have occurred, for the quick assignment of teams providing care, the medicines needed. It also educates on the basics in the alleviation of symptoms. Without a doubt, this will become a critical part of the library for any medical professional who attends to post-disaster crisis needs, whether at home or abroad."

—Alexandra Leigh, MD,
Section Chief of Hospice and Palliative Care,
Southeastern Louisiana Veterans Health Care System,
New Orleans, LA

"Waldman and Glass have courageously brought together multidisciplinary experts from both sectors to deliver this pioneering manual. *A Field Guide for Palliative Care in Humanitarian Crises* fundamentally recognizes that amidst dire humanitarian crises, palliative interventions need not be exhaustive or complex. Rather, attending to all dimensions of a person's illness experience through compassion, connection, ac-ceptance, and cultural humility should be at the heart of humanitarian palliative care efforts. This manual acknowledges that while we still have much to learn, there is a practical, moral, and legal imperative to alleviate suffering wherever it may be found. The *Field Guide* provides an essential platform upon which we can start."

—Rachel Coghlan, PhD Candidate,
Faculty of Arts and Education, Centre for Humanitarian Leadership,
Deakin University,
Victoria, Australia

A Field Manual for Palliative Care in Humanitarian Crises

Edited by

Elisha Waldman

Associate Professor of Pediatrics, Northwestern University
    Feinberg School of Medicine
Chief, Division of Palliative Care
Ann and Robert H. Lurie Children's Hospital of Chicago
Chicago, IL, USA

Marcia Glass

Associate Professor of Internal Medicine, Tulane University
    School of Medicine
Program Director, Tulane HPM Fellowship
New Orleans, LA, USA

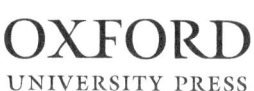

OXFORD
UNIVERSITY PRESS

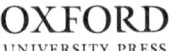

OXFORD
UNIVERSITY PRESS

Oxford University Press is a department of the University of Oxford. It furthers the University's objective of excellence in research, scholarship, and education by publishing worldwide. Oxford is a registered trade mark of Oxford University Press in the UK and certain other countries.

Published in the United States of America by Oxford University Press
198 Madison Avenue, New York, NY 10016, United States of America.

Library of Congress Control Number: 2019951720
ISBN 978–0–19–006652–9

This material is not intended to be, and should not be considered, a substitute for medical or other professional advice. Treatment for the conditions described in this material is highly dependent on the individual circumstances. And, while this material is designed to offer accurate information with respect to the subject matter covered and to be current as of the time it was written, research and knowledge about medical and health issues is constantly evolving and dose schedules for medications are being revised continually, with new side effects recognized and accounted for regularly. Readers must therefore always check the product information and clinical procedures with the most up-to-date published product information and data sheets provided by the manufacturers and the most recent codes of conduct and safety regulation. The publisher and the authors make no representations or warranties to readers, express or implied, as to the accuracy or completeness of this material. Without limiting the foregoing, the publisher and the authors make no representations or warranties as to the accuracy or efficacy of the drug dosages mentioned in the material. The authors and the publisher do not accept, and expressly disclaim, any responsibility for any liability, loss or risk that may be claimed or incurred as a consequence of the use and/or application of any of the contents of this material.

9 8 7 6 5 4 3 2 1

Printed by Marquis, Canada

Contents

Preface

Medical providers in resource-limited settings use many reference materials to look up diagnoses, epidemiology, and treatments. However, after working in settings around the world as palliative care physicians, we realized that there was no reference book written for clinicians working in crisis situations. Likewise, we acknowledged that, while deployment of palliative care specialty-trained clinicians with all humanitarian aid missions might seem like an admirable goal, the dearth of such clinicians makes attaining such a goal unlikely.

Thus, we recognized the need for a concise, practical manual that could be used by clinicians without palliative care training to incorporate principles of palliative care into their humanitarian work. We were fortunate enough to find a highly qualified, international group of palliative care specialists, internists, pediatricians, dermatologists, surgeons, therapists, chaplains, nurses, ethicists, lawyers, public health workers, palliative researchers, pain specialists, pharmacists, geriatricians, and emergency doctors with whom to collaborate. The end result is the manual that you hold in your hands.

We wrote this book with several possible audiences in mind. Most obviously, we wrote it for humanitarian aid workers who have no formal palliative care training. But we also wrote it for local providers to use for teaching and guidance in integrating palliative care into local relief efforts. Finally, we hope this manual will serve as a useful teaching tool in any educational setting for medical providers and trainees who may be called on one day to provide care in resource-limited and crisis settings.

We have covered the fundamentals of palliative care, including comprehensive symptom control, communication frameworks, and psychosocial support, with a particular focus on trauma-informed care. We have also built in public health material focused on the integration of palliative care into epidemics, conflicts, and natural disasters.

We hope this manual serves as an asset in the vital mission of alleviating the pain and suffering that may be experienced by people anywhere in the world facing humanitarian crises.

Acknowledgments

First and foremost, we'd like to thank all of those who have worked so hard over the years, and continue to work hard, dedicating themselves to the mission of helping people in need, wherever they are, and improving ongoing and future efforts. Without the work of so many, this manual would never have come about, particularly with the information so needed to serve those in crisis.

Thanks also go to Elizabeth Namukwaya and Mhoira Leng, who reviewed several chapters and welcomed many of our authors to Mulago Hospital as friends. Thanks go to the Médecins Sans Frontières (Doctors Without Borders; MSF) team, who sent some of us to the field, supported this book at various stages, and continue to provide life-saving services to those most in need all over the world. Thanks to the University of California at San Francisco (UCSF) Divisions of Palliative Care and Hospitalist Medicine, who not only trained many of us in the art of palliative care but also lent multiple authors to this project.

Additional thanks go to Tamar Amichai, Nicholas Coatsworth, Carrie Bernard, Elysee Nouvet, Matthew Hunt, and members of the Humanitarian Health Ethics Research Group, who shared their research and clinical experience, and to Catherine Habashy and Sarah Comolli, who contributed a pharmacological perspective to many chapters, in addition to their own.

And, finally, we owe thanks to our partners (Zach Lerner and Sasha Pick-Waldman), who understood how much we needed to do this, and to our parents, who inspired us to go.

Contributors

Tammam Aloudat, MD
Deputy Medical Director
Doctors Without Borders (MSF)
Geneva, Switzerland

Justin N. Baker, MD, FAAHPM
Chief, Division of Quality of Life and
    Palliative Care
Attending Physician, QoLA (Quality
    of Life for All) Team
Director, Hematology/Oncology
    Fellowship Program
St. Jude Children's Research Hospital
Memphis, TN, USA

**Susan Barbour, RN, MS, FNP,
    CWON, ACHPN**
Clinical Nurse Specialist in
    Palliative Care
University of California, San Francisco
    (UCSF) Medical Center
San Francisco, CA, USA

**Kevin Bezanson, MD,
CCFP(PC), DTMH, MPH**
Assistant Professor
Northern Ontario School of Medicine
Lakehead & Laurentian Universities
Thunder Bay, Ontario, Canada

Nahid Bhadelia, MD, MA
Assistant Professor of Medicine
Boston University School of Medicine
Medical Director, Special
    Pathogens Unit
National Emerging Infectious Diseases
    Laboratory
Boston, MA, USA

Lynn Black, MD, MPH
Instructor in Medicine
Harvard Medical School
Attending Physician, Department of
    Medicine
Massachusetts General Hospital
Boston, MA, USA
Chief Medical Officer
International Medical & Surgical
    Response Team
U.S. Department of Health and
    Human Services
Washington, DC, USA

**Peter Yuichi Clark, PhD,
MDiv, BCC**
Director of Spiritual Care Services for
    UCSF Health
University of California, San Francisco
San Francisco, CA, USA
Professor of Pastoral Care
American Baptist Seminary of
    the West at the Graduate
    Theological Union
Berkeley, CA, USA

Sarah L. Comolli, PharmD
Clinical Pharmacist, Adult Inpatient
    Pharmacy Services
Medical University of South Carolina
Charleston, SC, USA

Bethany-Rose Daubman, MD
Instructor in Medicine
Harvard Medical School
Attending Physician, Division of
    Palliative Care & Geriatrics
Massachusetts General Hospital
Boston, MA, USA

Megan Doherty, MD, FRCPC (Pediatrics)
Fellowship in Palliative Medicine
University of Ottawa
Children's Hospital of Eastern
    Ontario
Ottawa, Canada
Two Worlds Cancer Collaboration
Vancouver, Canada

Sandra L. Freiwald, MD, FACS
Southern California Permanente
    Medical Group–San Diego
Department of General Surgery
San Marcos, CA, USA

Stefan J. Friedrichsdorf, MD, FAAP
Children's Hospitals and Clinics of
    Minnesota
Department of Pediatrics, University
    of Minnesota
Minneapolis, MN, USA

Marcia Glass, MD
Associate Professor of Internal
    Medicine
Tulane University School of Medicine
Program Director, Tulane HPM
    Fellowship
New Orleans, LA, USA

Catherine Habashy, MD, MPH
Assistant Professor of Pediatrics
The George Washington University
    School of Medicine and Health
    Sciences
Attending Physician, Division of
    Hospitalist Medicine
Children's National Medical Center
Washington, DC, USA

Mara Haseltine, MD, FAAD
Clinical Assistant Professor of
    Dermatology
Tulane University School of Medicine
Department of Dermatology
New Orleans, LA, USA

Joshua Hauser, MD, FAAHPM
Northwestern Feinberg School of
    Medicine
Jesse Brown VA Medical Center
Chicago, IL, USA

Gary Hsin, MD, FAAHPM
Director, Hospice & Palliative
    Care Center
VA Palo Alto Health Care System
Clinical Associate Professor
    (Affiliated)
Stanford University School of
    Medicine
Palo Alto, CA, USA

Jessi Humphreys, MD
Assistant Professor of Palliative
    Medicine
Department of Medicine, Division of
    Palliative Medicine
University of California, San Francisco
San Francisco, CA, USA

Michaela Ibach, MD
Assistant Professor of Clinical
    Pediatrics
Division of Hospital Medicine, Section
    of Pediatric Palliative Care
Vanderbilt University Medical Center
Nashville, TN, USA

Sanja Janjanin, MD
Advisor for Anaesthesia &
    Critical Care
International Committee of the
    Red Cross
Geneva, Switzerland

Denah M. Joseph, BCC, MFT
Associate Chief for Wellness
University of California, San Francisco
Division of Palliative Medicine
Chaplain, UCSF Outpatient Palliative
    Care Clinic
San Francisco, CA, USA

Farzana Khan, MBBS, MPH, MA
President & CEO
Fasiuddin Khan Research Foundation
Dhaka, Bangladesh

Carrie Kovarik, MD
Associate Professor of Dermatology
  and Infectious Diseases
Departments of Dermatology and
  Medicine
Perelman School of Medicine at the
  University of Pennsylvania
Philadelphia, PA, USA

Eric L. Krakauer, MD, PhD
Associate Professor of Medicine
  and of Global Health & Social
  Medicine
Harvard Medical School
Director, Global Palliative Care
  Program
Massachusetts General Hospital
Boston, MA, USA
Honorary Chair, Department of
  Palliative Care
University of Medicine & Pharmacy at
  Ho Chi Minh City, Vietnam

**Mhoira E.F. Leng, FRCP
(Edinburgh and Glasgow)**
Palliative Care Specialist Physician
Senior Advisor
Makerere University Palliative Care
  Unit, Uganda
Chair of the Palliative Care
  Education and Research
  Consortium, Uganda
Medical Director
Cairdeas International Palliative Care
  Trust, Scotland
Senior Advisor, Global Health
  Academy
University of Edinburgh,
  Scotland

**Joan Marston, RN, B Soc Sc
(Hons), MA**
Co-founder and Co-chair
Palliative Care in Humanitarian
  Aid Situations and Emergencies
  (PalCHASE), hosted by the
  International Association for
  Hospice and Palliative Care
  (IAHPC)
Houston, TX, USA
Vice-chair
Palliative Treatment for Children
  (Patch), South Africa

**Stephanie Rogers, MD,
MS, MPH**
Assistant Professor of Medicine
Medical Director, Delirium Reduction
  Campaign
University of California, San Francisco
San Francisco, CA, USA

Sujatha Sankaran, MD
Associate Professor of Hospital
  Medicine
University of California, San Francisco
Division of Hospital Medicine
San Francisco, CA, USA

Lisa Schwartz, BA, MA, PhD
Professor, Arnold L. Johnson Chair in
  Health Care Ethics
McMaster University
Department of Health Research
  Methods, Evidence and
  Impact (HEI)
Hamilton, Ontario, Canada

Sriram Shamasunder, MD
Associate Professor of Hospital
  Medicine
University of California, San Francisco
Division of Hospital Medicine
San Francisco, CA, USA

Brett Sutton, MBBS, MPHTM, FAFPHM, FRSPH, FACTM, MFTM
Co-founder and Co-chair
Palliative Care in Humanitarian
 Aid Situations and Emergencies
 (PalCHASE), hosted by the
 International Association for
 Hospice and Palliative Care
 (IAHPC)
Houston, TX, USA
Chief Health Officer and Chief
 Human Biosecurity Officer
Victoria, Australia

Elisha Waldman
Associate Professor of Pediatrics,
 Northwestern University Feinberg
 School of Medicine
Chief, Division of Palliative Care
Ann and Robert H. Lurie Children's
 Hospital of Chicago
Chicago, IL, USA

Meaghann S. Weaver, MD, MPH, FAAP
Chief, Division of Pediatric
 Palliative Care
Children's Hospital and
 Medical Center
Omaha, NE, USA

David M. Williscroft, MD
Associate Clinical Professor
 in Emergency Medicine and
 Palliative Care
University of British Columbia
Attending Emergency Physician
Lions Gate Hospital
Consultant Palliative Medicine
 Physician
St. Paul's Hospital
Vancouver, British Columbia, Canada

Natasha Yacoub, LLM (Public International Law), LLB, BA (Hons)
Senior Legal Officer, Legal
 Protection Unit
United Nations High Commissioner
 for Refugees Regional
 Representation
Canberra, Australia

A Field Manual for Palliative Care in Humanitarian Crises

Chapter 1

Introduction

Why Palliative Care?

Elisha Waldman and Marcia Glass

Although humanitarian crises around the world show no signs of abating, and a number of factors, including climate change and recalcitrant conflicts, seem poised to continue driving and even increasing the frequency of crises in coming years, the scale and capability of international aid efforts has nonetheless grown with time. Humanitarian crises, defined by the World Health Organization (WHO) as "large-scale events that affect populations or societies causing a variety of difficult and distressing consequences that may include massive loss of life, disruption of livelihoods, breakdown of society, forced displacement, and other severe political, economic, social, psychological and spiritual effects,"[1] may take many forms, including natural disasters such as hurricanes and earthquakes, disease outbreaks (e.g., Ebola), and international refugee crises sparked by war, violence, or famine. Given this variety and complexity, it has become evident that international responses to crises must, to some extent, be tailored to the specific circumstances.

On a positive note, the scale and capability of international aid efforts have grown with time, and there is reason for hope with the ongoing improvement and increasingly effective responses from the international community. The number of humanitarian aid organizations continues to grow, and with time and experience operations continue to become more streamlined. Technology, especially the rise of social media, has allowed for rapid dissemination of information and real-time reporting, leading to an increased global awareness and rapid responses. Aid organizations also continue to make efforts at integrating responses with existing government and informal health structures and providers.

Another important development in healthcare in general offers an opportunity to improve services delivered during crises: the field of palliative care has grown from a small group of individuals interested in how to best care for the seriously ill and dying to a separate medical subspecialty with its own training and certification programs, focused on providing the best care possible to individuals and family members facing severe and life-limiting illness, regardless of how imminent death may be.

Recently, there has been increasing recognition of the importance of integrating palliative care into humanitarian aid. This is reflected in a growing number of journal articles and position papers on this topic, most notably the WHO publication *Integrating Palliative Care and Symptom Relief into the Response to Humanitarian Emergencies and Crises: A WHO Guide*, published in October 2018.

This increasing recognition is in part a reflection of the growth of palliative care as a medical subspecialty; it also reflects the increasing understanding that the goal of humanitarian aid is not simply to save lives, but also to alleviate suffering. This latter point cannot be overstated: when the primary focus of aid efforts remains simply and solely the saving of lives (which, of course, is a worthy goal), those efforts risk failing in the equally important, and morally and ethically compelling, goal of addressing suffering.

Additionally, there may well be a "trickle-up" effect—that is, by integrating principles of palliative care into the fundamental approach to all patients, starting from the moment of triage, overall care improves across the board, regardless of outcome. This includes better overall symptom management, better communication (between clinicians and patients and families as well as among clinicians themselves), and improved staff resilience. Simply put, integrating principles of palliative care into the care of all patients means better overall patient care and an improved healthcare system.

Currently, there are not enough formally trained and certified palliative care providers to staff every humanitarian aid mission in the world, nor does that solution make the most sense. Even in hospitals with robust palliative care teams, most emphasize educating other clinicians in primary palliative care skills as a way of amplifying treatment impact. In a similar fashion, we propose that while providers with advanced palliative care training would make a welcome addition to any humanitarian aid effort, the goal of widespread integration of palliative care into such efforts is more likely to succeed through the training of aid workers in principles of primary palliative care that they can themselves apply, regardless of whether clinicians with more advanced training are present. This manual is intended to be a first step toward providing clinicians without formal palliative care training the guidance and education required for addressing basic palliative care needs while responding to humanitarian crises.

The manual is divided into three sections. The first section deals with conceptual issues around integrating palliative care into humanitarian crises—what that might look like and in what ways integration must be tailored to the specific crisis. The second section deals with specific symptoms or symptom clusters—for example, how to manage dyspnea in someone with severe injury or progressive disease, or how to manage symptoms in an actively dying patient. Finally, the third section addresses psychosocial issues such as grief and self-care.

The manual is intended to be above all else *practical*. Each chapter is designed to be lean and focused, putting practical information at the clinician's fingertips. It is *not* intended to act as a foundational textbook on any of the topics it covers. In addition, while we hope that this manual may prove useful to local clinicians trying to provide palliative care in the context of humanitarian crises, we must acknowledge that this manual was written by clinicians from higher economic–status countries. It is worth recognizing at the outset that while this approach has its advantages, it also leads to some shortcomings. These shortcomings may be most pronounced in the psychosocial chapters (Chapters 16–17), where discussions of how to provide culturally sensitive and appropriate care for every possible setting is simply beyond the scope of this manual. Clearly, issues like providing support around grieving and bereavement are heavily culture dependent. As noted in these later chapters, we encourage incorporating local providers for these purposes wherever possible. But for the purposes of this manual, we focus on how providers in the midst of challenging and often overwhelming situations can best begin incorporating principles of palliative care. Given the fraught conditions in which these providers work, we have embedded the theme of trauma-informed care throughout the book.

There remains much work to be done in this field. We hope to some day see better research on the topics covered here, more comprehensive textbooks, and more formalized training programs to optimize the integration of palliative care into humanitarian relief efforts. In the meanwhile, we hope that this manual provides some useful, practical guidance for those undertaking this incredibly important work.

Reference

1. World Health Organization. *Integrating Palliative Care and Symptom Relief into the Response to Humanitarian Emergencies and Crises: A WHO Guide.* Geneva: World Health Organization; 2018.

Chapter 2

Palliative Care Needs of People Affected by Natural Hazards, Political or Ethnic Conflict, Epidemics of Life-Threatening Infections, and Other Humanitarian Crises

Eric L. Krakauer, Bethany-Rose Daubman, Tammam Aloudat, Nahid Bhadelia, Lynn Black, Sanja Janjanin, and Farzana Khan

Introduction

Traditionally, humanitarian healthcare response has focused primarily on saving lives and has lacked a concerted focus on preventing and relieving suffering. Yet the principles of humanitarianism explicitly require prevention and alleviation of human suffering,[1,2] and the imperative of saving lives does not conflict with the imperative of relieving suffering in most situations.[3] Patients deemed "expectant" (expected to die) often suffer severely before they die, and failure to endeavor to relieve their suffering constitutes unethical abandonment (see Chapter 15). During comfort-oriented care, triage should be repeated because it may reveal that a patient deemed expectant could be saved, either because the patient's condition unexpectedly stabilizes or because additional life-saving resources arrive. Humanitarian crises may be triggered by natural hazards (earthquakes, major storms, tsunamis, floods, droughts), violent political or ethnic conflict, epidemics of life-threatening infections, release of radiation, or other disastrous events. However, humanitarian crises rarely are caused by a single factor and are usually the result of mixed natural, human-made, environmental, political and economic causes and vulnerabilities.[3] The consequences may vary greatly depending on the causes, location, and vulnerability of the population they affect, but the consequences often include extensive loss of life and physical, psychological, social, and spiritual suffering on a massive scale (Table 2.1). The poor, the displaced (refugees and internally displaced persons), and those living in low-income settings generally are most vulnerable to unnecessary suffering and death because healthcare and social support systems in their areas may be weak, dysfunctional, inaccessible, unaffordable, overburdened, or destroyed.

Table 2.1. Common Symptoms and Forms of Distress Caused Directly by Humanitarian Emergencies*

	Ebola Epidemic	Earthquake	Genocide/War	Influenza Pandemic[†]
Pain	X	X	X	X
Dyspnea	X	X		X
Nausea/vomiting	X			
Diarrhea	X			
Fever	X			X
Fatigue/weakness	X			
Delirium	X			
Cough	X			X
Dizziness	X			
Conjunctivitis	X			
Oedema	X			
Acute stress reactions	X	X	X	X
PTSD	ND	X	X	
Other anxiety disorders	X	X	X	
Depressive symptoms	ND	X	X	
Stigmatized/social isolation	X			X
Complicated grief	ND			X

ND, no data; PTSD, post-traumatic stress disorder.

*Light gray indicates acute symptoms or distress, medium gray indicates chronic symptoms or distress, and dark gray indicates acute or chronic symptoms or distress, or both. † Hypothetical.

Sources: WHO (2018);[2] Leong et al. (2004);[3] Rieder and Elbert (2013);[5] MacNeil et al. (2010);[6] Schieffelin et al. (2014);[7] Dallatomasina et al. (2015);[8] Mollica et al. (2004);[9] Angeletti et al. (2012);[10] Downar and Seccareccia (2010);[11] Roy et al. (2005);[12] Wu et al. (2014);[13] Kristensen et al. (2012);[14] Li et al. (2015);[15] Caffo and Belaise (2003);[16] Catani et al. (2008);[17] West and von Saint André-von Arnim (2014);[18] Teodorescu et al. (2015).[19]

Natural Hazards: Earthquakes, Major Storms, Tsunamis, Floods

Sudden-onset disasters due to natural hazards commonly cause suffering and death on a large scale and also may devastate the social and medical infrastructure needed to care for the sick and injured (Table 2.2). In these situations, palliative care is needed:

1. By patients actively dying from acute injury;
2. By patients who may live for days or weeks with injuries or illnesses that are nonsurvivable in a disaster context or who develop nonsurvivable complications;
3. By patients not in immediate danger of dying but with moderate or severe symptoms;
4. By patients with pre-existing serious illness, disability, or frailty who have lost access to healthcare;[20–22]
5. By family members of patients with any of the preceding conditions; and
6. By the severely psychologically traumatized or socially vulnerable.

In the immediate aftermath, surgical and life-sustaining resources often are inadequate to the need.[23] However, emergency medical teams (EMTs) always should be equipped to provide palliative care. The essential package of palliative care medicines and equipment needed for safe and effective symptom control is small and inexpensive (see Chapter 13),[3] and WHO has published model guidelines to enable transport of controlled medicines such as morphine across international borders for emergency medical care.[24] Governments and humanitarian organizations also should help ensure that local healthcare providers in hospitals and in the community have adequate palliative care training and supplies, particularly in areas most at risk for sudden-onset disasters.

Earthquakes

Earthquakes commonly cause collapse of buildings with resultant crush injuries and associated symptoms of pain, dyspnea, and psychological trauma, among others. Immediate and ongoing pain relief and psychological support should accompany surgical, critical, and rehabilitative care. Many rescued victims of earthquakes die weeks later of complications, such as local or systemic infection related to wounds, renal failure due to rhabdomyolysis, or sequelae of lacking food, shelter, or medicine for chronic conditions. Patients may suffer from any number of physical and psychological symptoms depending on their specific medical, psychological, and social situation.

Tsunamis

Tsunamis often cause both traumatic injuries and health problems distinct from those caused by other natural hazards.[25,26] These include the following:

- Aspiration pneumonitis
- Respiratory infections, often with rare or drug-resistant pathogens
- Respiratory failure due to pneumonitis or infection

Table 2.2. Types of Suffering of People Affected by Sudden-Onset Disasters, War, Political Conflict, or Ethnic Violence and Recommended Steps to Integrate Palliative Care into Humanitarian Responses

Type of Suffering	Recommended Palliative Care Responses to Suffering
Physical Suffering	
Symptoms due to acute injury or illness Symptoms due to injury-related complications and subacute or chronic illnesses	• Put in place policies clarifying that humanitarian medical assistance aims to both save lives and relieve suffering • Develop protocols for a minimum standard of symptom assessment and treatment, and for care of expectant patients, by international and national emergency medical teams (EMTs) and local healthcare providers. • Train and equip EMTs and local healthcare providers to reach a minimum standard of symptom assessment and treatment and care of expectant patients. • Include the essential package of palliative care medicines and equipment for humanitarian emergencies and crises in all emergency health kits; ensure that oral and injectable morphine are included in all kits and are both secured and accessible in adequate quantities by EMTs and local healthcare providers. • Include in all type 1 EMTs at least one physician and nurse with at least basic palliative care training. • Include in all type 2 and 3 EMTs at least one physician with at least intermediate palliative care training and that all anesthetists and anesthesia technicians have at least basic palliative care training.
Psychological Suffering	
Acute psychological effects (including acute anxiety, acute depressed mood, acute grief) Chronic psychological effects (including PTSD, chronic anxiety disorders, chronic depression, complicated grief, survivor's guilt, substance use disorders)	• Train EMT staff members and local healthcare providers in psychological first aid (PFA) • Train and equip EMTs and local healthcare providers with protocols for psychological symptom assessment and treatment • Include the essential package of palliative care medicines and equipment for humanitarian emergencies and crises in all emergency health kits; include oral fluoxetine, injectable diazepam, and oral and injectable haloperidol in all kits so that they are accessible in adequate quantities to EMTs and local healthcare providers.[21] • Train and equip all EMTs in palliative care as described earlier. • Seek partnerships with local community and spiritual leaders for advice on cultural values and beliefs relevant to mental illness and to inform the local community about the EMTs' activities. • Recruit local mental health care providers who can provide culturally and linguistically appropriate care and advise foreign team members on cultural values and beliefs relevant to mental illness.

(continued)

Table 2.2. Continued	
Type of Suffering	**Recommended Palliative Care Responses to Suffering**
	• Offer training to local volunteers to provide basic mental health interventions as appropriate.
	• Organize support groups for patients and survivors who may wish to share experiences and challenges.
	• Include mental health care providers in humanitarian response teams that are likely to encounter many patients with mental health consequences.
Social Suffering	
Loss of access to shelter, clothing, food, sanitation, protection from violence, school (for children)	• Ensure access to shelter, clothing appropriate to climate and culture, food, sanitation, school.
	• Seek to arrange protection from physical or psychological abuse.
Extreme vulnerability (including frail older people, unaccompanied children, people with mental or physical disabilities, people living in extreme poverty)	• Organize support groups for patients and survivors who may wish to share experiences and challenges.
Spiritual Suffering	
Loss of sense of meaning of life	• Seek partnerships with local spiritual counselors willing to visit patients and family members on request.
Loss of faith or angry with God	

Sources: WHO (2018).[3] Adapted from IASC (2007);[28] Smith and Aloudat (2017);[29] Knaul et al. (2018);[30] Krakauer (2018).[31]

• Soft-tissue infections with rare or drug-resistant pathogens

• Tetanus

Integrated critical care and palliative care is needed for patients with respiratory failure or tetanus.

Major Storms and Floods

Major storms and floods may not only destroy or incapacitate healthcare facilities but also cut them off from resupply. Hospitals and long-term care centers in areas commonly affected by storms and floods should have evacuation plans in place, a backup generator, and at least a 10-day supply of oxygen, food and water, basic antibiotics, essential medicines for noncommunicable diseases, and all items that constitute the essential package of palliative care (see Chapter 13).[3,22]

War, Political Conflict, and Ethnic Violence

War, political conflict, and ethnic violence commonly cause many types of suffering on a vast scale due to injuries (Table 2.2).[27] Beyond acute physical and psychological trauma, destruction of local infrastructure and services and mass displacement can result in exposure to still more violence and to harsh climates. These conditions also may result in malnutrition and in infectious outbreaks among the population. Often, most displaced persons are women, children, and older adults, who are especially vulnerable to exploitation, sexual abuse, rape, and torture.[32]

Pain should be treated aggressively in any patient. Acute and chronic anxiety, depression, post-traumatic stress disorder (PTSD, and complicated grief are common sequelae that humanitarian responders should be prepared to diagnose and treat (Table 2.1). Basic training in mental health and psychosocial support (MHPSS) should be included in palliative care training for humanitarian responders, as it equips them to provide focused, nonspecialized psychological support, such as psychological first aid (PFA) and treatment of uncomplicated adjustment disorder and mood disorders, for affected persons and for responders.[33] Psychiatrists and psychologists can be helpful in planning and implementing specialized mental health care for affected persons and responders.[28] Spiritual counselors with experience in palliative care or disaster response also can be helpful in planning and implementing psychological and spiritual support (Table 2.2).

Epidemics of Life-Threatening Infections

During epidemics of life-threatening infections, suffering may result from both the disease and the medical or public health response. Thus, it is important to train EMTs and local healthcare providers to anticipate adverse effects of treatment and to apply preventative measures as appropriate.

Disease symptoms vary depending on the infection (Table 2.1). Some epidemic infections result in physical, psychological, social, and spiritual suffering. Physical symptoms of Ebola infection typically include nausea, vomiting, diarrhea, body aches, fever, and, in late stages, bleeding, respiratory distress, and encephalopathy.[34] Aggressive control of nausea, vomiting, and diarrhea not only relieves unnecessary suffering but also can protect against volume depletion and electrolyte derangements and hence may improve survival. It also can reduce contamination of enclosed, shared spaces within Ebola treatment units with virus-laden body fluids, hence lessening the risk of transmission to healthcare workers. In some widespread life-threatening infections, such as multidrug-resistant tuberculosis, adverse reactions to treatment commonly cause significant suffering and make adherence to treatment difficult.[35] Thus, pain and symptom control is crucial for a variety of reasons.[3]

Quarantine of people exposed to an epidemic life-threatening infection and isolation of those with active infection may be necessary from a public health perspective. However, the benefits and harms should be considered carefully because quarantine and isolation typically exacerbate psychological and social suffering.[28,36] Quarantined and isolated patients often feel anxious, sad, and dehumanized. Thus, patients' time in isolation wards should be kept to the minimum time necessary for infection control, and the wards should be organized to enable patients to communicate with family members and friends at a distance or with mobile phones. Patients should be informed regularly about their condition and prognosis in a way appropriate for their culture and education and literacy level. Voluntary psychosocial support groups can be organized for patients, survivors, and bereaved family members, psychosocial supporters, local spiritual counselors, and mental health staff members should receive infection control training and equipment necessary to safely visit infected patients. Psychosocial supports should remain accessible to survivors and family members (especially orphans) who may continue to suffer from mental health problems, stigmatization, social isolation, and extreme poverty.[37] Community education can be conducted to reduce fear and stigma and improve infection control, and community reintegration programs for survivors can be organized with community or religious leaders.

Nuclear Detonation

A nuclear war would result in sudden and prolonged suffering and death on an unprecedented scale owing to physical and psychological trauma, burns, radiation sickness, epidemic disease, starvation, and exposure to the elements. Thus, all healthcare providers should advocate intensively for abolition of nuclear weapons and prevention of war.[38] To advocate effectively, and to prepare to respond as effectively as possible to this suffering, it is important to anticipate what specific needs would arise. Acute radiation syndrome (ARS) typically involves three phases. The duration of each depends on the total radiation dose and the rate at which it is delivered. After initial radiation exposure there may be a prodromal phase, with symptoms such as nausea, vomiting, and lethargy. During the latent phase, a person feels relatively well before developing the phase of organ system dysfunction. The organ systems most susceptible to radiation injury are, in order of vulnerability, the hematological system, the gastrointestinal tract, the skin, and cerebrovascular system. Patients who receive a high level of exposure typically develop severe organ system failure, have a very poor prognosis, and should receive comfort-oriented care.[39] The psychological trauma of a nuclear detonation may result in acute stress disorder, PTSD, anxiety disorders, major depression, complicated bereavement, unexplained physical symptoms, sleep disturbance, family conflict and violence, and substance use disorders.[40]

Triage

Regardless of the types of humanitarian crisis or the types of suffering it causes, several principles apply to the triage process (Table 2.3):

1. Palliative care and life-saving treatment should not be regarded as distinct. Palliative care should be integrated as much as possible with life-saving treatment for patients with acute life-threatening conditions (triaged red).

2. Palliative care must be provided for all patients deemed expectant (triaged blue) and should commence immediately.[41]

3. Palliative care should commence immediately, as needed, for patients with non-life-threatening conditions whose injury- or disease-specific treatment may be delayed (triaged yellow).

Table 2.3. Recommended Triage Categories in Humanitarian Emergencies and Crises

Category	Color Code	Description
1. Immediate	Red	Survival possible with immediate treatment.
		Palliative care should be integrated with life-sustaining treatment as much as possible.
2. Expectant	Blue	Survival not possible given the care that is available.
		Palliative care is required.
3. Delayed	Yellow	Not in immediate danger of death, but treatment needed soon.
		Palliative care and/or symptom relief may be needed immediately.
4. Minimal	Green	Will need medical care at some point after patients with more critical conditions have been treated.
		Symptom relief may be needed.

Source: WHO (2018).[3]

4. Repeat triage should be practiced, especially for patients triaged blue and yellow, to make sure that important changes in the patient's condition that should result in a change in triage category are not missed.

References

1. International Committee of the Red Cross (ICRC). *Fundamental Principles of the Red Cross and Red Crescent Movement.* Geneva: International Committee of the Red Cross (ICRC); 1986. https://www.icrc.org/en/fundamental-principles. Accessed June 23, 2019.

2. Sphere Association. *The Sphere Handbook: Humanitarian Charter and Minimum Standards in Humanitarian Response*, 4th ed. Geneva: Sphere Association; 2018. https://www.spherestandards.org/handbook. Accessed June 23, 2019.

3. World Health Organization (WHO). *Integrating Palliative Care & Symptom Relief into Responses to Humanitarian Emergencies & Crises: A WHO Guide.* Geneva: World Health Organization; 2018.

4. Leong IY, Lee AO, Ng TW, et al. The challenge of providing holistic care in a viral epidemic: opportunities for palliative care. *Palliat Med.* 2004;18:12–18.

5. Rieder H, Elbert T. The relationship between organized violence, family violence and mental health: findings from a community-based survey in Muhanga, Southern Rwanda. *Eur J Psychotraumatol.* 2013;4.

6. MacNeil A, Farnon EC, Wamala J, et al. Proportion of deaths and clinical features in Bundibugyo Ebola virus infection. *Uganda Emerg Infect Dis.* 2010;16:1969–1672.

7. Schieffelin JS, Shaffer JG, Goba A, et al. and the KGH Lassa Fever Program; Viral Hemorrhagic Fever Consortium; WHO Clinical Response Team. Clinical illness and outcomes in patients with Ebola in Sierra Leone. *N Engl J Med.* 2014;371:2092–2100.

8. Dallatomasina S, Crestani R, Sylvester Squire J, et al. Ebola outbreak in rural West Africa: epidemiology, clinical features and outcomes. *Trop Med Int Health.* 2015;20:448–454.

9. Mollica RF, Cardozo BL, Osofsky HJ, et al. Mental health in complex emergencies. *Lancet.* 2004;364:2058–2067.

10. Angeletti C, Guetti C, Papola R, et al. Pain after earthquake. *Scand J Trauma Resusc Emerg Med.* 2012;20:43. doi:10.1186/1757-7241-20-43

11. Downar J, Seccareccia D, Associated Medical Services Inc. Palliating a pandemic: "All patients must be cared for". *J Pain Symptom Manage.* 2010;39:291–295.

12. Roy N, Shah H, Patel V, Bagalkote H. Surgical and psychosocial outcomes in the rural injured: a follow-up study of the 2001 earthquake victims. *Injury.* 2005;36:927–934.

13. Wu Z, Xu J, He L. Psychological consequences and associated risk factors among adult survivors of the 2008 Wenchuan earthquake. *BMC Psychiatry.* 2014;14:126.

14. Kristensen P, Weisæth L, Heir T. Bereavement and mental health after sudden and violent losses: a review. *Psychiatry.* 2012;75:76–97.

15. Li J, Chow AY, Shi Z, Chan CL. Prevalence and risk factors of complicated grief among Sichuan earthquake survivors. *J Affect Disord.* 2015;175:218–223.

16. Caffo E, Belaise C. Psychological aspects of traumatic injury in children and adolescents. *Child Adolesc Psychiatr Clin N Am.* 2003;12:493–535.

17. Catani C, Jacob N, Schauer E, et al. Family violence, war, and natural disasters: a study of the effect of extreme stress on children's mental health in Sri Lanka. *BMC Psychiatry.* 2008;8:33.

18. West TE, von Saint André-von Arnim A. Clinical presentation and management of severe Ebola virus disease. *Ann Am Thorac Soc.* 2014;11:1341–1350.

19. Teodorescu DS, Heir T, Siqveland J, et al. Chronic pain in multi-traumatized outpatients with a refugee background resettled in Norway: a cross-sectional study. *BMC Psychol.* 2015;3:7.

20. Wilkinson A. The potential role for palliative care in mass casualty events. *J Palliat Care Med.* 2012;2:e112.

21. Karunakara U, Stevenson F. Ending neglect of older people in the response to humanitarian emergencies. *PLoS Med.* 2012;9(12):e1001357.

22. Slama S, Kim HJ, Roglic G, et al. Care of non-communicable diseases in emergencies. *Lancet.* 2017; 389:326–330.

23. Goodman A, Black L. The challenge of allocating scarce medical resources during a disaster in a low income country. *Palliat Med Hosp Care Open J.* 2015;1:24–29.

24. World Health Organization (WHO). *Model Guidelines for the International Provision of Controlled Medicines for Emergency Medical Care.* Geneva: World Health Organization; 1996. http://apps.who.int/medicinedocs/en/d/Jwho32e/. Accessed June 23, 2019.

25. Guha-Sapri D, van Panhuis WG. Health impact of the 2004 Andaman Nicobar earthquake and tsunami in Indonesia. *Prehosp Disaster Med.* 2009;24:493–499.

26. Doocy S, Robinson C, Moodie C, Burnham G. Tsunami-related injury in Aceh Province, Indonesia. *Global Pub Health.* 2009;4:205–214.

27. Matzo M, Wilkinson A, Lynn J, Gatto M, Phillips S. Palliative care considerations in mass casualty events with scarce resources. *Biosecur Bioterror.* 2009;7:199–210.

28. Inter-Agency Standing Committee. *IASC Guidelines for Mental Health and Psychosocial Support in Emergency Settings.* Geneva: Inter-Agency Standing Committee Geneva (IASC); 2007.

29. Smith J, Aloudat T. Palliative care in humanitarian medicine. *Palliat Med.* 2017;31(2):99–101. doi:10.1177/0269216316686258

30. Knaul FM, Farmer PE, Krakauer EL, et al. Alleviating the access abyss in palliative care and pain relief: an imperative of universal health coverage. *Lancet.* 2018;391:1391–1454.

31. Krakauer EL, Kwete X, Verguet S, et al. Palliative care and pain control. In: Jamison DT, Gelband H, Horton S, et al., eds. *Disease Control Priorities*, 3rd ed. Vol. 9: *Improving Health and Reducing Poverty.* Washington DC: World Bank; 2018:235–246.

32. Pedersen D. Political violence, ethnic conflict, and contemporary wars: broad implications for health and social well-being. *Social Science & Medicine.* 2002;55(2):175–190.

33. World Health Organization (WHO). *mhGAP Humanitarian Intervention Guide: Clinical Management of Mental, Neurological and Substance Use Conditions in Humanitarian Emergencies.* Geneva: World Health Organization; 2015. http://www.who.int/mental_health/publications/mhgap_hig/en/. Accessed June 23, 2019.

34. Bah EI, Lamah MC, Fletcher T, et al. Clinical presentation of patients with Ebola virus disease in Conakry, Guinea. *N Engl J Med.* 2015;372:40–47.

35. Awofeso N. Anti-tuberculosis medication side-effects constitute major factor for poor adherence to tuberculosis treatment. *Bull World Health.* 2008;86(3):B–D.

36 Pellecchia U, Crestani R, Decroo T, et al. Social consequences of Ebola containment measures in Liberia. *PLoS One.* 2015;10(12):e0143036.

37. Van Bortel T, Basnayake A, Wurie F, et al. Psychosocial effects of an Ebola outbreak at individual, community and international levels. *Bull World Health.* 2016;94:210–214.

38. Helfand I, Sidel VW. Docs and nukes—Still a live issue. *N Engl J Med.* 373;20:1901–1903.

39. Coleman CN, Weinstock DM, Casagrande R, et al. Triage and treatment tools for use in a scarce resources—crisis standards of care setting after a nuclear detonation. *Disaster Med Public Health Prep.* 2011;5:S111–S121.

40. Dodgen D, Norwood AE, Becker SM, et al. Social, psychological and behavioral responses to a nuclear detonation in a US city: implications for health care planning and delivery. *Disaster Med Public Health Prep.* 2011;5:S54–S64.

41. World Health Organization (WHO), International Committee of the Red Cross (IARC). WHO/ICRC Technical Meeting for Global Consensus on Triage; 2017. https://www.humanitarianresponse.info/sites/www.humanitarianresponse.info/files/documents/files/triage_2017_meeting_report-b.pdf. Accessed June 23, 2019.

Chapter 3

Practical Tips on Integrating Palliative Care

Brett Sutton and Joan Marston

Introduction

Ensuring the integration of palliative care into healthcare responses to humanitarian crises varies depending on the type of crisis and length of time that aid is required. Humanitarian crises take myriad forms and thus can be extremely variable in length and complexity. The average length of crises with an active inter-agency appeal rose from 4 to 7 years between 2005 and 2017,[1] reflecting the increasing complexity and protracted nature of current crises. There is, therefore, a real need to respond to rapidly emergent or short-term crises while recognizing that the overall trend is increasing numbers and increasingly likely to be protracted.[1]

Providing palliative care requires organizational policies, guidelines, and standards that include palliative care; training, education, and skills; access to essential palliative care equipment and medicines, including opioids; collaboration and integration with local services; and close engagement and support of palliative care specialists.

The Sphere Standards and the Cluster System

All acute crises require palliative care expertise to be integrated into the initial or existing healthcare response.

The foundational standards for coordination and collaboration are set out in the *Sphere Handbook,* specifically Core Standard 2, which provides guidance on the actions required to ensure that coordination and collaboration are embedded in an agency's response. Such standards apply for UN or non-UN agencies, and international as well as regional or local responders. These key actions within this standard include such aspects as participation; sharing of agency mandate; information sharing in the response; policy on and practice in engagement; and being informed about the coordination role of the state and other coordination groups.[2] In addition, the *Sphere Handbook* outlines in Standard 2.6, Care of Non-communicable Diseases, the need to establish a referral system, including to palliative and supportive care. Finally, the 2018 edition of the *Sphere Handbook* incorporates—for the first time—a specific standard on palliative care. This is essential reading for anyone providing or intending to provide palliative care in humanitarian settings, as it lays out key actions that support integration. These include the establishment of guidelines and policies, including for triage; development of care plans; integration at all levels of the health system, focusing on home-based care; training of healthcare workers; and working closely with local systems and networks.[2]

This last key action—working with local systems—is critically important to ensure that patients, caregivers, and families are supported in the community and at home. Such local systems may include national palliative care associations, hospices, faith-based organizations, and local medical and nonmedical staff experienced in palliative care in the country.

One essential mechanism for the coordination of agencies in emergencies is the cluster system was proposed by the IASC (Inter-Agency Standing Committee) of the UN in 2006 to improve humanitarian effectiveness. Clusters comprise humanitarian organizations across the main sectors in emergencies. For palliative care, the relevant cluster is health, and the global cluster lead is the World Health Organization (WHO), often co-chaired with a national government representative.[3]

Localization and the National Disaster Management Office

Coming out of the World Humanitarian Summit in 2016, there was much focus on the issue of localization, to meet the growing global humanitarian challenge. But as the Australian Red Cross has noted, "the dominant approach to localisation within organisations has been to tweak—in a programmatic sense—rather than re-think the systematic approach to local humanitarian action."[4]

In researching this issue, the Pacific region provided a definition (now adopted by the Organisation for Economic Co-operation and Development [OECD][5]) of localization as ". . . a process of recognising, respecting and strengthening the independence of leadership and decision making by national actors in humanitarian action, in order to better address the needs of affected populations." Recommendations arising from this research highlighted key requirements for effective localized action, including leadership by national actors at all levels; building on and strengthening local practices; maximizing national and regional capacity before requesting international support; and being directed by nationally appropriate tools, systems, and processes.

In integrating palliative care to strengthen the formal healthcare system and attain long-term sustainability, these key approaches must be explicitly considered and used. One essential point of engagement in-country will be the National Disaster Management Office (NDMO) or its equivalent. The NDMO is the national coordinating agency for disasters within a country and must be engaged with for any responding individual or organization. The NDMO will be constituted differently by country but has a leading role and must be respected as the sovereign decision-making body regarding deployments to areas of need and the prioritization of activities and affected populations. Any responders must contact the NDMO and ensure that they engage with the cluster approach, if in operation.[3]

Emergency Medical Teams

Emergency medical teams (EMTs) are groups of health professionals providing medical care locally and internationally in humanitarian emergencies. Their work is supported by WHO-established minimum standards and a global registry.

While the WHO classification of EMTs is focused on surgical care, in general terms it has a "sliding scale" of care from EMT type 1 to type 3, with EMT type 3 being most complex and specialized. An EMT type 1 provides outpatient emergency care, EMT type 2 provides inpatient surgical emergency and other general care, and EMT type 3 provides complex inpatient referral surgical care including intensive care.

Palliative care clinicians would likely be deployed in an EMT type 3, but palliative care services can and should be considered for all EMTs by ensuring the competencies, essential medications, and guidance are integrated at all levels.[3]

Foundations for Integration of Palliative Care

The existing evidence base regarding integration of palliative care into emergency humanitarian settings is currently limited. There is, however, evidence of effective integration into longer-term humanitarian situations in Jordan,[6] Bangladesh,[7] Nepal,[8] and Uganda.[9]

There is also evidence of successful palliative care integration in low-resource settings. Malawi, for example, has a national palliative care policy and a national development program for adults and children. There is also enormous palliative care experience and expertise that has been developed through the well-documented response to HIV, AIDS, and tuberculosis in sub-Saharan Africa[10] that should be drawn on in responding to humanitarian crises locally and internationally. Based on this expertise the following elements comprise a foundation of palliative care integration:

- Inclusion of palliative care in organizational policy of humanitarian healthcare response teams, locally and internationally

- Routine or "just-in-time" training of humanitarian healthcare workers in all essential components of palliative care provision

- Routine or "just-in-time" training of palliative care specialist teams or individuals regarding working in humanitarian situations[3]

- Training of community-based palliative care providers in basic palliative care surveillance, counseling, and spiritual and psychosocial support

- Embedding the principles of localization by maximizing the capacity of local health services and giving leading roles to existing care organizations and networks[4]

- Ensuring that existing or newly established referral pathways for patients requiring specialist care include palliative care[11]

- Routine surveillance to identify palliative care needs, involving community members[11]

- An embedded referral system involving both nongovernmental and government organizations

- Access to palliative care medicines, including opioids, incorporated into local systems of pharmaceutical storage, distribution, prescription, and provision[11]

- Provision of palliative care beds in hospitals and clinics, if feasible

Integrating Palliative Care into Long-Term Humanitarian Emergencies

Many acute emergencies, particularly complex humanitarian emergencies, can become protracted, and agencies must therefore look at ways to integrate palliative care fully within routine care provision for affected populations, akin to development contexts.

Such integration can occur through:

- Building palliative care expertise across primary healthcare staff. This requires training of all providers in the principles and practice of palliative care.

- Inclusion of a palliative care team or specialists within the primary healthcare system. Palliative care expertise can be made available for direct care, in an advisory capacity, or to facilitate referral out of the humanitarian areas, if available.[11]

- Training, mentoring, and supervision of community members as palliative care assistants and volunteers,[9] utilizing technology for training, communication, and expert advice.[12]

- Provision of independent palliative care teams through an external agency or from within the country[8]

- Establishment of a palliative care centre linked to a community palliative care team or teams[9]

Ultimately, integration of palliative care into the local healthcare system is a longer-term objective, in line with the Sustainable Development Goal of universal health coverage.[13]

References

1. United Nations Office for the Coordination of Humanitarian Affairs (OCHA). World Humanitarian Data and Trends. 2018. https://data.humdata.org/dataset/world-humanitarian-data-and-trends. Accessed February 9, 2019.

2. Sphere Association. *The Sphere Handbook: Humanitarian Charter and Minimum Standards in Humanitarian Response*, 4th ed. Geneva: Sphere Association; 2018. https://ww.spherestandards.org/handbook. Accessed June 23, 2019.

3. World Health Organization (WHO). *Integrating Palliative Care and Symptom Relief into the Response to Humanitarian Emergencies and Crises: a WHO Guide*. Geneva: World Health Organization; 2018. Licence: CC BY-NC-SA 3.0 IGO.

4. Ayobi Y, Black A, Kenni L, Nakabea R, Sutton K. Going Local: Achieving a More Appropriate and Fit-for-Purpose Humanitarian Ecosystem in the Pacific. October 2017. https://www.redcross.org.au/getmedia/fa37f8eb-51e7-4ecd-ba2f-d1587574d6d5/ARC-Localisation-report-Electronic-301017.pdf.aspx. Accessed June 24, 2019.

5. Organisation for Economic Co-operation and Development (OECD). Localising the Response. World Humanitarian Summit: Putting Policy into Practice 2017. https://www.oecd.org/development/humanitarian-donors/docs/Localisingtheresponse.pdf. Accessed June 24, 2019.

6. Pinheiro I, Jaff D. The role of palliative care in addressing the health needs of Syrian refugees in Jordan. *Med Confl Surviv*. 2018; 34(1):1–20.

7. Doherty M, Khan F. Neglected suffering. The Unmet Need for Palliative Care in Cox's Bazaar. World Child Cancer; 2018. https://reliefweb.int/

report/bangladesh/neglected-suffering-unmet-need-palliative-care-cox-s-bazar. Accessed June 24, 2019.

8. Munday D, Basnyat R, Swarbrick E, et al. Palliative care in Nepal: current steps to providing universal health coverage. *Eur J Palliat Care*. 2018;25(1):40–46.

9. Integrating Palliative Care into Humanitarian Contexts in Uganda: A Health Systems Strengthening Approach. Hospice Africa Uganda. 2018.

10. Inter-Agency Standing Committee. Guidelines for Addressing HIV in Humanitarian Settings. UNAIDS; 2010. https://www.unaids.org/sites/default/files/media_asset/jc1767_iasc_doc_en_0.pdf. Accessed June 24, 2019.

11. UNICEF, Division of Communication. *Core Commitments for Children in Humanitarian Action*. New York: UNICEF; 2010.

12. World Health Organization (WHO). *WHO Compendium of Innovative Health Technologies for Low-Resourced Settings*. Geneva: World Health Organization; 2016-2017.

13. Gómez-Baptiste X, Connor S, et al. The foundations of palliative care public health programs. In: Gómez-Baptiste X, Connor S, eds. *Building Integrated Palliative Care Programs and Services*. Catalonia: 2017.

Chapter 4

Pain Management

Elisha Waldman and Stefan J. Friedrichsdorf

Introduction

Although palliative care involves much more than just pain treatment, effective analgesia is nonetheless a critical part of such care. This will be an adjunct to management of the underlying condition, regardless of whether definitive treatment is available or not, and is also essential in the management of acute trauma. In fact, if pain is not well managed, it may not be possible to determine the underlying condition added to the devastating impact of unrelieved acute and chronic pain on the individual, family, and healthcare workers. As noted in earlier chapters, appropriate pain treatment and alleviation of suffering should be viewed as a human right and as part of any comprehensive care plan, regardless of likelihood of survival.

Pain may be roughly categorized as acute, chronic, acute-on-chronic, or procedural. Chronic pain may also be classified as a subtype of pain that travels through undamaged pain pathways (nociceptive) and through damaged pathways (neuropathic). Beyond the scope of this chapter (but discussed in Chapter 16) is also the concept of total pain and various types of emotional, psychological, and existential suffering; assessment and management of the holistic needs of a person and family are nonetheless essential. Indeed, in a post-trauma situation it may be that physical chronic pain has causes that are strongly related to the nonphysical trauma, and both must be addressed. Thus assessment must include awareness of social, cultural, psychological, and spiritual issues, including awareness of mental health needs and the roles that fear, anxiety, and exposure to violence, such as rape or witnessing killing, may have on the experience and expression of pain.

Pain management and palliative care require a multidisciplinary approach. As noted in elsewhere in this manual, whenever possible, local resources for pain management as well as for psychosocial support should be identified and included in planning and management of the healthcare response.

Proper pain treatment requires first and foremost access to necessary medications and equipment. These are covered in Chapter 13 in this book. In addition to having the means for treating pain at hand, in order to arrive at an appropriate treatment plan it is also important, through careful history-taking and examination, to identify the degree and type of pain a patient may be experiencing. This may be especially challenging in the context of a humanitarian crisis, where there may be significant language and cultural barriers and it may be difficult to discern chronic from acute pain.

Regardless of the type of pain and the likelihood of patient survival, in order to achieve ongoing control of pain, clinicians should strive to arrive at a carefully considered individualized pain plan that may involve a combination of medications as well as integrative (nonpharmacological) interventions.

Pain Assessment

Assessing the type and degree of pain is of course easiest when one is faced with a calm, oriented, and verbal patient. In such a situation through careful history-taking and examination one may quickly arrive at an assessment of pain needs. Careful attention should be paid to nonverbal cues, such as facial expression, body position, and vital signs. This pain history will include the site of the pain (there may be several), the severity, how the pain moves, when it comes on, what words are used to describe the pain such as burning or stabbing, and anything that help relieves the pain or makes it better. To aid assessment a number of report measures have been widely validated to help gauge the severity of the pain and pain relief. Some of the more detailed formats, such as the Brief Pain Inventory questionnaire, may be impractical in emergency situations. More widely used are visual analogue scales (commonly used with both adults and children) or numerical rating scales, for example rating one's pain on a scale from 0 to 10 with 10 being the worst pain imaginable.

Infants and small children, as well as nonverbal adults, are at particular risk for underappreciation and undertreatment of pain (see Chapter 12). When possible, parents or caregivers who know the child should be asked for their sense of a child's pain. In addition, for neonates, infants, or children with neurological impairment one may use the Revised-Face, Leg, Activity, Cry, Consolability (r-FLACC) scale.

Multidimensional Observational Rating Scales

For nonverbal patients and children younger than 4 years, pain is measured using observation rating scales. Examples include the following:

• **Infants**: Infant FLACC scale (see Table 4.1)[1]
• **Toddlers, older nonverbal children**: FLACC pain scale (0–10)[2]
• **Nonverbal, intellectually impaired persons**: r-FLACC (see Box 4.1)[3]

Self-Assessment

• **4- to 6-year-olds**: Simplified Faces Pain Scale (S-FPS) or Simplified Concrete Ordinal Scale (S-COS) (see Fig. 4.1)[4]
• **6- to 12-year-olds**: Faces Pain Scale–revised (see Fig. 4.2)[5]
• **Individuals >10 years of age**: Visual Analogue Scale (VAS) (see Fig. 4.3)[6] or Numerical Rating Scale (NRS-11) (see Fig. 4.4)[7]

Assessment should, of course, be an ongoing undertaking, and patients, regardless of triage status, should be regularly re-evaluated for improvement or worsening of pain and the impact of any interventions.

Table 4.1. Infant FLACC Scale

Infant FLACC Scale

Category	Scoring		
Face	No particular expression or smile	Occasional grimace or frown, withdrawn, disinterested	Frequent to constant quivering chin, clenched jaw
Legs	Normal position or relaxed	Uneasy, restless, tense	Kicking or legs drawn up
Activity	Lying quietly, normal position, moves easily	Squirming, shifting back and forth, tense	Arched, rigid, or jerking
Cry	No cry (awake or asleep)	Moans or whimpers, occasional complaint	Crying steadily, screams or sobs, frequent complaints
Consolability	Content, relaxed	Reassured by occasional touching, hugging or being talked to, distracted	Difficult to console or comfort

Instructions: Each of the five categories is scored from 0 to 2, which results in a total score between 0 and 10.
Source: From Merkel, Voepel-Lewis, and Malviya (2002).

Treatment of Pain

Having assessed the pain, one may formulate an individualized pain plan for a given patient. A plan should include selection of appropriate medications with an appropriate administration schedule, selection of an appropriate route, and on-going re-evaluation and adjustment as dictated by the patient's needs. Although this may sound self-evident, the principles laid out here are critical for achieving

Box 4.1 Revised FLACC Observational Pain Tool for Pain Assessment in Children with Cognitive Impairment

Face

0 = No particular expression or smile
1 = Occasional grimace/frown; withdrawn or disinterested; *appears sad or worried*
2 = Consistent grimace or frown; frequent/constant quivering chin, clenched jaw; *distressed-looking face; expression of fright or panic*
Individualized behavior: _____

Legs

0 = Normal position or relaxed; *usual tone and motion to limbs*
1 = Kicking, or legs drawn up; *marked increase in spasticity, constant tremors or jerking*
Individualized behavior: _____

From Malviya et al. (2006). © Wiley. Reprinted with permission.

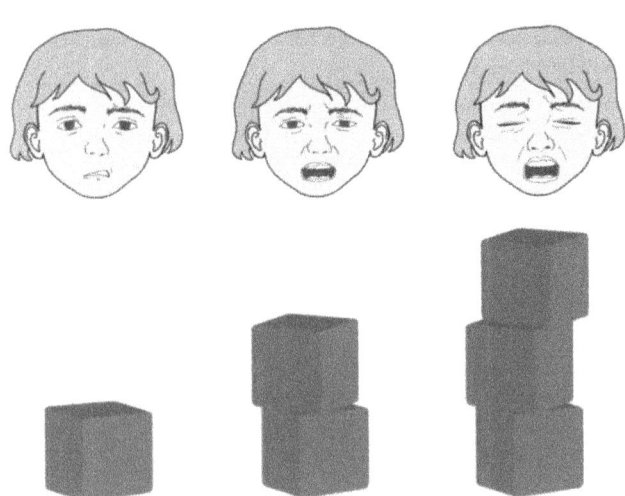

Figure 4.1. Simplified Faces Pain Scale (S-FPS) or Simplified Concrete Ordinal Scale (S-COS) for 4- to 6-year-old children. Instructions: Ask the child whether or not they are in pain. If yes, show faces or building blocks to evaluate for "mild," "medium," or "severe" pain. (Reprinted from Emmott, West, et al., 2017, with permission from Elsevier.)

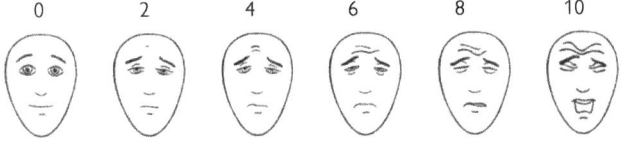

Figure 4.2. Faces Pain Scale–Revised (FPS-R) for children age 7 years and older. The instructions, and translations into more than 60 languages, are available at: http://www.iasp-pain.org/Education/Content.aspx?ItemNumber=1519. (Reprinted with permission from Hicks, von Baeyer, et al., 2001.)

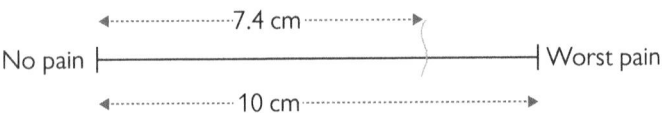

Figure 4.3. Visual Analogue Scale (VAS). (Reprinted with permission from Bailey, Gravel, et al., 2012.)

No Pain 0 1 2 3 4 5 6 7 8 9 10 *Worst Pain*

Figure 4.4. Numerical Rating Scale (NRS-11). (Reprinted with permission from von Baeyer, Spagrud, et al., 2009.)

good pain control; pain management cannot be viewed as a one-time, one-dose procedure.

Route and timing are important issues. Some medications may be available only in intravenous or enteral forms, and, conversely, some patients may be unable to take enteral or intravenous forms. Thus careful consideration must be given in choosing enteral (oral, sublingual, rectal), intravenous, subcutaneous, or topical or transdermal routes.

In addition, medications should not be given as one-time doses. The aim is to keep the patient pain-free regardless of whether the pain is acute or chronic. To do this, medications should be prescribed "by the clock" or by regular administration (e.g., oral morphine is normally scheduled every 4 hours) with frequent re-evaluation and titration as dictated by the clinical situation. As-needed (PRN) orders alone (i.e., without scheduled analgesia) cannot be recommended, as the end result is often that no medication is given at all. However, PRN medication may be scheduled *in addition to* the regular dose, to manage rescue or breakthrough pain, which is pain occurring in between the regular dosing. This dose can be calculated in different ways, but a simple way is to use the following formula, which works for both children and adults:

Example: for a child (10 kg) with severe acute pain: Oral morphine 0.3 mg × 10 kg = 3 mg every 4 hours. Additional breakthrough (PRN or "rescue" dose) would be 10% of the daily total dose (3 mg every 4 hours = 18 mg/day), or 1.8 mg every 1–2 hours as needed.

For a detailed list of essential medications, along with routes and dosing, please see Chapter 13. In general, pain medications can be divided into three classes: nonopioids, opioids, and adjuvants. In addition, we will briefly touch on here integrative and nonpharmacological therapies. It is important to note that good pain management usually requires a combination of approaches, particularly when the pain is severe. Regardless of type and quality of pain, a rational, stepwise approach to managing pain, including escalation of dosage and class of drug when necessary, is central to quality care (see Box 4.2 at the end of the chapter for a sample algorithm).

Basic Analgesics

This category includes paracetamol (acetaminophen), ibuprofen, and other non-steroidal anti-inflammatory drugs (NSAIDs), which may be suitable for milder pain. These agents also play a role in conjunction with opioids for more severe pain and may provide additional benefits depending on the clinical scenario, such as antipyretic activity.

Opioid Analgesics

This category includes weak opioids such as tramadol as well as strong opioids such as morphine, fentanyl, hydromorphone, and methadone. Codeine, a weak opioid and a prodrug in its administered form, is no longer widely used because

Box 4.2 Pain Management Algorithm

Step 1: Conduct pain assessment (see Chapter 4 for further details).

Step 2a: Mild to moderate pain (initial dose)

- **PARACETAMOL**
  Route: PO/PR/IV
  Adult Dose: 500 mg q4–6h
  Pediatric Dose: 15 mg/kg/dose (15–20 mg/kg PR) q4h

and/or

- **IBUPROFEN**
  Route: PO
  Adult Dose: 400–800 mg q6h (max 3.2 g/day)
  Pediatric Dose: 10 mg/kg/dose q6h (max 40 mg/kg/day)

or

- **DICLOFENAC**
  Route: PO
  Adult Dose: 50 mg q8–12h
  Pediatric Dose: 1 mg/kg/day divided bid or tid

Step 2b: Moderate to severe pain (initial dose)

- **MORPHINE** (preferred when available)
  Route: PO/SL/PR/IV/SC
  Adult Dose:
- PO/SL/PR: 5–15 mg q4–6h
- IV/SC: 2–5 mg q2–4h
  Pediatric Dose:
- PO/SL/PR: 0.15–0.3 mg/kg/dose q4–6h
- IV/SC: 0.05–0.15 mg/kg/dose q2–4h

or

- **TRAMADOL** (if morphine or other strong or standard opioid is not available)
  Route: PO
  Adult Dose: 50–100 mg q4–6h
  Pediatric Dose (4–16 years): 1–2 mg/kg/dose q4–6h

and

- **PARACETAMOL, IBUPROFEN, or DICLOFENAC** (dosing in Step 2a)

Step 3: Assess response. If analgesia is effective, continue medicine on scheduled basis ("around the clock"). If ineffective, continue to Step 4.

Step 4a: Mild to moderate pain (ineffective analgesia with initial treatment)
- If pain is uncontrolled on a single agent, add a second agent (paracetamol or NSAID).
- Consider trial of a different NSAID class (ibuprofen vs. diclofenac).
- If there is no improvement, switch to moderate to severe pain algorithm (Step 2b).

Step 4b: Moderate to severe pain (ineffective analgesia with initial treatment)
- If ineffective analgesia with morphine, increase dose by 50% and assess response.
- Continue to titrate dose by 50% every third dose until analgesia is reached or signs of sedation occur.
- *Respiratory depression is rare with appropriate dose escalation.*
- If analgesia is achieved but subsequently lost after stable dosing, evaluate for new or worsening sources of pain. Also consider development of tolerance and opioid rotation if alternate opioids are available.

Step 5: Address other considerations for pain syndromes not responsive to initial therapies

- Pain due to muscle spasm (e.g., fractures, chronic contractures)
  - Add **DIAZEPAM**

    Route: PO/SL/buccal/PR/IV

    Adult Dose:
    - PO: 2–10 mg q6–8h
    - IV: 2–10 mg q3–4h

    Pediatric Dose:
    - PO: 0.04–0.3 mg/kg/dose q6–8h
    - IV: 0.04–0.3 mg/kg/dose q3–4h

- Neuropathic pain (e.g., diabetic neuropathy, HIV neuropathy)
  - Add **AMITRIPTYLINE**

    Route: PO

    Adult Dose: 25 mg qhs, titrate to 100 mg qhs

    Pediatric Dose: 0.1 mg/kg/dose qhs, titrate to 0.5–2 mg/kg/dose qhs

    or

  - Add **GABAPENTIN**

    Route: PO

    Adult Dose: Initial dose 100–300 mg 1 to 3 times daily; increase to target range of 300–1200 mg 3 times daily

    Pediatric Dose: Initial dose 10–15 mg/kg/day in 3 divided doses; titrate as tolerated to effective dose

- Bone pain
  - Add **DEXAMETHASONE**

    Route: PO/SL/PR/IM/IV

    Adult Dose: 4 mg q8–12 h

    Pediatric Dose: 0.15 mg/kg/dose q8–12h

    Start GI prophylaxis with ranitidine or omeprazole.

- Anxiety exacerbating pain-related distress
  - Add **LORAZEPAM**

    Route: PO/SL/PR/IM/SC/IV

    Adult Dose: 0.5–2 mg q8h

    Pediatric Dose: 0.05 mg/kg/dose q4–8h (max 2 mg, max starting dose 0.5 mg)

    or

  - Add **DIAZEPAM**

    Route: PO/SL/buccal/PR/IV

    Adult Dose:
    - PO: 2–10 mg q6–8h
    - IV: 2–10 mg q3–4h

    Pediatric Dose:
    - PO: 0.04–0.3 mg/kg/dose q6–8h
    - IV: 0.04–0.3 mg/kg/dose q3–4h

bid, twice daily; GI, gastrointestinal; IM, intramuscular; IV, intravenous; NSAID, nonsteroidal anti-inflammatory drug; PO, oral; PR, rectal; qhs, every bedtime; SC, subcutaneous; SL, sublingual; tid, three times daily.

of concerns about unpredictable metabolism leading to both undertreatment and unexpected adverse events. We would therefore recommend against its use, although, of course, if this is the only agent available and there are no other options, clinicians may exercise judgment based on the clinical setting.

The choice of opioid may depend heavily on availability. In general, if there is a clinical suspicion of renal impairment, fentanyl or methadone may be preferable, owing to concerns about toxic accumulation of metabolites of morphine and hydromorphone in this setting. If morphine or hydromorphone are used in the setting of renal failure, clinicians should remain alert to the risk of metabolites building up, leading to myoclonus (often misinterpreted as discomfort) and seizures.

Other side effects of opioids that clinicians should remain aware of and that may complicate the clinical picture are constipation and drowsiness (which tends to pass after the first day or so, and often represents patients simply catching up on sleep now that their pain is being adequately managed). Urinary retention may also be observed at times, which may necessitate placement of a urinary catheter. Concern about any of these side effects is NOT a reason to avoid use of opioids, as pain management is of paramount importance and can be effective and safe using the guidelines as given.

Individuals differ in their response to opioid analgesics. If patients with serious illnesses treated for pain or dyspnea display opioid-induced side effects, such as oversedation, *and* experience good symptom control, then it might be reasonable to reduce the opioid dose. If, however, both poor analgesia and dose-limiting side effects occur, opioid rotation has been shown to be very effective to improve analgesia and dyspnea management and to lessen side effects.[8,9] Differences between opioids in the balance between analgesic cross-tolerance level and the level of cross-tolerance to adverse effects can be exploited to clinical advantage. If opioids are being rotated because of decreasing effectiveness or limiting side effects (i.e., because of incomplete cross-tolerance), it is best to begin at around 50% of the equianalgesic dose and titrate to effect. However, the required decrease for incomplete cross-tolerance may be higher or lower, depending on the clinical context of the individual patient.[10] For clinicians inexperienced in opioid rotation, we suggest reaching out, when possible, to available colleagues with pain and anesthesia training for guidance.

Adjuvant Medications and Interventions

Adjuvant medications are used mostly in combination with basic analgesics and opioids for specific pain types in order to maximize analgesia. They are sometimes used alone, but are often helpful as opioid-sparing agents, especially when there is a neuropathic component to the pain. Circumstances in which these medications may be particularly helpful include the following:

1. Neuropathic pain such as herpes zoster or peripheral nerve damage
2. Muscle spasm affecting abdominal organs (smooth muscle) or back pain (skeletal muscle)

3. Pressure cause by inflammation or tumors that affect organs and nerves, such as raised intracranial pressure, liver capsule stretch, or tumors pressing on nerves

Adjuvants include tricyclic antidepressants such as amitriptyline (or nortriptyline) and the anticonvulsant gabapentin (or pregabalin). Generally speaking, these agents tend to be useful when there are neuropathic components to the pain. These medication may take days to weeks to show effect and in combination are usually more effective than alone.

NMDA receptor antagonists may also play a role as adjuvant medications. Methadone, which acts both as an opioid and as an NMDA antagonist, may be especially useful because of the dual mechanism. Ketamine is an agent in this category that may be useful in the context of procedural pain or as an adjuvant medication when given in low (subanesthetic) doses.

Corticosteroids of any sort may be useful as adjuncts in the management of pain, in particular bony pain or headaches due to increased intracranial pressure. Corticosteroids, of course, have a number of common and well-known side effects, often limiting their longer-term use.

Integrative (Nonpharmacological) Treatment Modalities

Integrative modalities (sometimes referred to as *complementary or alternative medicine*) that have been described as effective in the management of pain include hypnosis, yoga, acupuncture, and massage. Active mind–body techniques, such as guided imagery, hypnosis, biofeedback, yoga, and distraction, all evoke pain modulation by engaging a number of mechanisms within the analgesic neuraxis.

Relaxation therapy might include progressive muscle relaxation to help patients recognize and lower body tension associated with pain and anxiety. Patients can be taught how to tense and relax different muscle groups in a relaxed and quiet setting, or to visualize a happy or peaceful scene and reduce body tensions. Breathing techniques such as patterned, shallow, or deep breathing can be used alongside relaxation approaches.

Hypnosis involves the cultivation of an altered state of awareness, leading to heightened suggestibility that allows for changes in perception and experience, bypassing conscious effort.[11] In hypnosis the clinician enters the patient's world, engaging the patient's imagination as the agent of change and creating alternate experiences to promote therapeutic change. In trance, the patient addresses distressing symptoms utilizing suggestions by the clinician for altering sensations and perceptions and increasing comfort.[12] Teaching hypnosis to patients, even to children and adolescents, is an extremely versatile skill, which can be acquired by clinicians through formalized training workshops and practice.[13]

Other cognitive and behavioral methods that may have a particular role in the care of children include comfort measures such as pacifiers, massage, touch, and music; distraction methods such as bubbles, counting, toys, and video games; and suggestion methods such as magic glove or magic blanket techniques.

Procedural Pain and Regional Anesthesia

Procedural anesthesia lies beyond the scope of this manual, though it should be remembered that any procedure, even one done in the context of palliative measures (e.g., pleurocentesis) should be accompanied by some sort of analgesia. Regional blocks may also play an important role in pain management, especially if the condition is likely terminal or in an acute trauma setting (e.g., pelvic or extremity tumor, severe extremity crush injury). Anesthesiologists and pain specialists accompanying a humanitarian aid mission may be unaware of the potential applications of their skills in the context of palliative care; providers should therefore make every effort to reach out to and integrate those specialists into the care of patients with palliative needs.

Care of the Dying Patient

Care of the dying patient is covered in detail in Chapter 9. Pain and symptom management is an important component of the care plan for dying patients. It should be remembered that opioids are the gold standard for management of pain and/or dyspnea, and that sedation may mask the symptoms (by inducing sleep or coma) but does not actually address the symptoms. Sedative agents such as benzodiazepines may well play a role in the management of patients with severe pain who are dying or otherwise, but these should not be confused with analgesic agents and proper pain management.

References

1. Merkel S, Voepel-Lewis T, Malviya S. Pain assessment in infants and young children: the FLACC scale. *Am J Nurs*. 2002;102(10):55–58.

2. Willis MH, Merkel SI, Voepel-Lewis T, Malviya S. FLACC Behavioral Pain Assessment Scale: a comparison with the child's self-report. *Pediatr Nurs*. 2003;29(3):195–198.

3. Malviya S, Voepel-Lewis T, Burke C, Merkel S, Tait AR. The revised FLACC observational pain tool: improved reliability and validity for pain assessment in children with cognitive impairment. *Paediatr Anaesth*. 2006;16(3):258–265.

4. Emmott AS, West N, Zhou G, et al. Validity of simplified versus standard self-report measures of pain intensity in preschool-aged children undergoing venipuncture. *J Pain*. 2017;18(5):564–573.

5. Hicks CL, von Baeyer CL, Spafford PA, van Korlaar I, Goodenough B. The Faces Pain Scale–revised: toward a common metric in pediatric pain measurement. *Pain*. 2001;93(2):173–183.

6. Bailey B, Gravel J, Daoust R. Reliability of the visual analog scale in children with acute pain in the emergency department. *Pain*. 2012;153(4):839–842.

7. von Baeyer CL, Spagrud LJ, McCormick JC, Choo E, Neville K, Connelly MA. Three new datasets supporting use of the Numerical Rating Scale (NRS-11) for children's self-reports of pain intensity. *Pain*. 2009;143(3):223–227.

8. Drake R, Longworth J, Collins JJ. Opioid rotation in children with cancer. *J Palliat Med*. 2004;7(3):419–422.

9. Fine PG, Portnoy RK; Ad Hoc Expert Panel on Evidence Review and Guidelines for Opioid Rotation. Establishing "best practices" for opioid rotation. *J Pain Symptom Manage*. 2009;38(3):418–425.

10. Friedrichsdorf SJ, Postier A. Management of breakthrough pain in children with cancer. *J Pain Res*. 2014;7:117–123.

11. Friedrichsdorf SJ, Kohen DP. Integration of hypnosis into pediatric palliative care. *Ann Palliat Med*. 2018;7(1):136–150.

12. Kohen DP, Olness KN. *Hypnosis and Hypnotherapy with Children*. New York: Routledge Publications, Taylor & Francis; 2011.

13. National Pediatric Hypnosis Training Institute (NPHTI). http://www.nphti.org. Accessed June 25, 2019.

14. World_Health_Organization (WHO). *WHO Principles of Acute Pain Management for Children*. Geneva: World Health Organization; 2012. http://whqlibdoc.who. int/publications/2012/9789241548120_Guidelines.pdf.

Chapter 5

Dyspnea

Meaghann S. Weaver

Definition

Dyspnea or breathlessness is the subjective experience of breathing discomfort. Dyspnea is a common end-of-life symptom for adults and for children, warranting palliative care attentiveness to the suffering associated with a sense of air hunger or a feeling of suffocation.

Measurement

A patient with normal blood gas, normal respiratory rate, and normal oxygen saturation level may still be experiencing dyspnea. Given the subjective nature of dyspnea, dyspnea is measured by patient report. Dyspnea can be measured using tools (such as the Edmonton Symptom Assessment Scale, Dalhousie Dyspnea Scale, Cancer Dyspnea Scale, or standard numerical scales) sequentially. For patients who are not able to self-report their extent of dyspnea, owing to developmental status or inability to express, close monitoring of nonverbal signs or distress observation scales can be considered.

Treatment

Consider interventions to target the underlying medical condition that may be causing the dyspnea if these are within the goals of care. Examples include use of bronchodilators or inhaled steroids for chronic obstructive pulmonary disease (COPD), use of transfusions for anemia, use of diuretics or angiotensin-converting enzyme (ACE) inhibitors or inotropes in congestive heart failure (CHF), use of cancer-directed therapies for lung tumor, use of antibiotics for pneumonia, and use of a tunneled drainage catheter for pleural effusion.

Steps and considerations in treating dyspnea include the following:

- Reposition the patient to positions of comfort; consider elevating the chest with pillow support.
- Circulate air via open windows or blowing fans with the goal of keeping air flowing.
- Teach pursed-lip meditation breathing: inhale peacefulness and calm slowly via the nose; exhale stress and fear via pursed lips.
- Consider supplemental oxygen for comfort.

- Avoid smoke exposure and avoid wearing strong fragrances.
- Reduce secretions with pharmaceuticals such as atropine drops under the tongue or scheduled anticholinergics, offer gentle suctioning, and avoid overly thickening secretions.
- Foster a calm environment, as anxiety symptoms worsen breathlessness, and the sense of air hunger worsens anxious feelings.
- Noninvasive ventilator support may be considered in certain diagnoses according to the goals of care.
- Honor family presence and relaxation for the family members and for the patient.
- Consider gentle wind-instrument music as background noise in the room for the comfort of surrounding the senses with the reminder of a breezy, refreshing air.

Pharmaceuticals Interventions

Opioids are the preferred approach to symptomatically treating dyspnea (see Table 5.1).

For an opioid-naïve adolescent or adult patient, consider starting 5 mg morphine equivalent by mouth or sublingual dose every 4 hours as needed for dyspnea. The dose may be decreased and the frequency extended if the patient seems too sedated; likewise, the dose may be increased by 25–50% or the frequency may be shortened to every 1 hour for severe, persistent dyspnea. For an opioid-naïve child or elderly patient, consider starting the morphine dose at half the above-recommended dose.

For patients who are actively dying and experiencing end-of-life dyspnea, consider a long-acting form of opiate for dyspnea, a continuous infusion of opiate, or a scheduled short-acting opiate.

Respiratory depression is almost always proceeded by drowsiness. One can consider a "hold for sedation" order when prescribing opiates for dyspnea.

A benzodiazepine such as lorazepam or diazepam may be considered as an anxiolytic if the patient is experiencing anxiety associated with shortness of breath.

A corticosteroid may be considered if the dyspnea is associated with COPD, lymphangitis, or asthma.

A bronchodilator may be added if bronchospasm is present.

Education

The patient, family, and staff should receive caring communication about the goal of dyspnea management, which is to manage the symptom of dyspnea, not to hasten death.

Provision of parameters for safe dosing of opiates for dyspnea, continual staff reassessment of the patient's response to dyspnea interventions, and open communication regarding the goals of symptom management are encouraged.

Table 5.1. PCHC Dyspnea Algorithm

Step 1: Assess dyspnea on the basis of patient report or standardized scale.

Step 2: Treat underlying conditions when feasible and appropriate for goals of care.

Step 3: Implement nonpharmacological interventions.

• Reposition patient to position of comfort, elevate chest.

• Circulate air: open windows, use fans.

• Consider supplemental oxygen for hypoxemic patients.

Step 4: Treat dyspnea with opioid analgesic.

• MORPHINE
Route: PO/SL/PR/IV/SC
Adult Dose:
  • PO/SL/PR: 5–15 mg q4–6h
  • IV/SC: 2–5 mg q2–4h
    • Decrease dose by 50% if patient is elderly or renal disease is present.
Pediatric Dose:
  • PO/SL/PR: 0.15–0.3 mg/kg/dose q4–6h
  • IV/SC: 0.05–0.15 mg/kg/dose q2–4h

Step 5: Evaluate response (using method used in Step 1). If dose is ineffective, increase by 25–50%. If there is excess sedation, decrease dose by 25–50%.

Step 6: Once effective dose and interval are established, schedule as needed or around the clock (may need to give as frequently as every hour at end of life.)

Step 7: Consider addition of benzodiazepine if anxiety is contributing to dyspnea.

• LORAZEPAM (preferred)
Route: PO/SL/PR/SC/IV
Adult Dose: 0.5–2 mg q8h
    • Decrease dose by 50% if patient is elderly or liver disease is present.
Pediatric Dose: 0.05 mg/kg/dose q4–8h (max 2 mg, max starting dose 0.5 mg)

or

• DIAZEPAM
Route: PO/SL/buccal/PR/IV
Adult Dose:
  • PO: 2–10 mg q6–8h
  • IV: 2–10 mg q3–4h
    • Decrease dose by 50% if patient is elderly or liver disease is present.
Pediatric Dose:
  • PO: 0.04–0.3 mg/kg/dose q6–8h
  • IV: 0.04–0.3 mg/kg/dose q3–4h

IV, intravenous; PO, oral; PR, rectal; SC, subcutaneous; SL, sublingual.

Dyspnea is holistically addressed by considering the patient's entire discomfort profile, including spiritual, psychological, and relational care needs in addition to physical needs.

Chapter 6

Gastrointestinal Symptom Management

Gary Hsin

Diarrhea

Overview

Diarrhea is defined as passage of loose or watery stool, typically with at least three episodes in 24 hours.[1] It is further classified as acute, lasting 14 days or less; persistent, lasting 15–30 days; and chronic, which continues for more than 30 days.[2] In resource-limited settings, the cause is most likely an infectious agent. Antimicrobials are not always warranted but may be necessary, especially in situations such as diarrhea due to *Shigella* infection or severe cholera.

Common causes of diarrhea include the following:

- Overflow due to impaction from either severe constipation or colorectal tumors
- Side effect of medications or anti-cancer treatment such as chemotherapy and radiotherapy
- Malabsorption due to prior surgeries such as resections or pancreatic insufficiencies
- Neuroendocrine (NE) tumors, for example, Zollinger-Ellison syndrome

Management

In a palliative care context, it is important to rule out constipation and impaction. Clinicians should consider using point-of-care ultrasound (POCUS) for assessment if available. If the diarrhea is due to an obstructive process, then surgical intervention may be necessary for either resection or diversion if this is a viable option. For patients with rectal or other obstructive tumors in whom surgery is not possible, the goal is to produce very soft stools with aggressive laxative use so that they can easily pass around the tumor.

Sanitation and infection control are of paramount importance, especially in situations where people are living in close quarters (e.g., refugee camps). Rehydration is an important component of care in palliation, and guidelines should be followed; however, in terminally ill patients this may lead to volume overload and should be used carefully for comfort when needed, or not at all in certain circumstances, such as with active dying. For all bedbound patients, good perineal skin care is especially important.

Pharmacological Management

Following are guidelines for pharmacological management of gastrointestinal (GI) symptoms (see Chapter 13 for additional dosing guidelines):

- Appropriate antibiotics should be given, if needed, based on local infection patterns. Use antimotility agents with caution in patients with infectious etiology.
- Antisecretory and antimotility agents such as glycopyrrolate, loperamide, or diphenoxylate-atropine are typically used as first-line medications.
  - Glycopyrrolate 1–2 mg PO qd–tid PRN; 0.1–0.4 mg IV/SC qd–tid
  - Loperamide 4 mg PO followed by 2 mg for each subsequent loose stool up to 16 mg/day
  - Diphenoxylate-atropine 5 mg qd–qid up to 20 mg/day
- Somatostatin analog: For refractory diarrhea or diarrhea due to chemotherapy or NE tumors, octreotide can be helpful and effective.
  - Octreotide 100–150 mcg SC/IV q8h up to 500 mcg q8h
- Bulking agents (fiber): In certain patients, dietary soluble fibers such as psyllium or methylcellulose can be of help; however, patients must be able to maintain adequate fluid intake.

Constipation

Overview

Constipation is typically characterized by infrequent and difficult defecation, often with painful passage of hard, small stool. This is a very common problem for frail, elderly, critically ill, and terminally ill patients and can have a significant impact on patients' quality of life. Severe constipation may lead to overflow diarrhea, urinary retention, delirium, nausea, and vomiting.

Common causes of constipation include the following:

- Poor diet in disaster and conflict zones
- Dehydration and immobility
- Disease of the GI tract
  - Cancers, strictures, fissures, proctitis
- Metabolic disturbances
  - Hypothyroid, hypercalcemia, hypokalemia, diabetes, paraneoplastic syndrome
- Neurological disorders
  - Spinal cord injury, malignant spinal cord compression, parkinsonism
- Medications
  - Opioids, antiemetics (e.g., $5HT_3$ inhibitors, prochlorperazine), anticholinergics, cardiovascular medications, psychiatric medications, supplements (e.g., iron and calcium)

Management

The performance of a rectal examination for rectal tone, fecal impaction, fissures, hemorrhoids, enlarged prostate, tumors, and other issues is critical. Plain film, ultrasound, and other imaging are usually unnecessary. Underlying medical and surgical issues should be addressed. When necessary, manual disimpaction should be performed.

In general, patients should be encouraged to increase mobility whenever possible and to consume a diet conducive to regular bowel movements. It is important to maintain adequate hydration, especially if osmotic agents are being used. Fiber-based bulking agents such as psyllium and cellulose may result in worsening constipation if the patient is unable to consume sufficient water. Docusate, which is a "surfactant/detergent laxative," has very questionable efficacy with little to no evidence base—in addition, the liquid tastes horrible.

Patients with an ostomy may require a bowel regimen to avoid constipation. Rectal suppositories are generally still effective for patients with a colostomy, since their rectal circulation and innervation are still intact. Rectal stimulation may be required for patients with a spinal cord injury or some other neurogenic cause for constipation. Patients who have minimal or no oral intake will continue to make small amounts of stool from sloughing of intestinal luminal cells and gut bacteria.

Pharmacological Management

Following are guidelines for pharmacological management of constipation (see Chapter 13 and Box 13.1 for dosing guidelines).

Patients typically need both an osmotic agent to provide softening and lubrication and neurostimulation for promotility kinetic effect, commonly referred to as "mush and push." Neurostimulants act as promotility agents by providing direct stimulation of the lower GI plexus to induce peristalsis and propulsion. Orally administered senna and bisacodyl are activated and absorbed in the colon (lower GI) in 6–12 hours and have little to no stimulant effect on the stomach (gastroparesis) or small intestines. Rectal formulations (suppositories or enemas) act much faster. Suppositories are rapidly converted by rectal flora to their active form in approximately 15–60 minutes. The most common side effect is abdominal cramping.

Osmotic agents play an important role by providing lubrication and softening, and they help trigger stretch receptors in the GI tract. Polyethylene glycol-3350 (PEG-3350) is an iso-osmotic polymer, which makes it very safe to use, especially for maintenance, even for children, the elderly, and the very ill. It easily dissolves into any kind of liquid at any temperature but does require patients to drink 200 mL or more to be effective. As a dose-dependent agent, it can be rapidly acting when given in large volumes.

Sugar-based laxatives include lactulose, sorbitol, and mannitol. They work mainly in the colon by drawing in water and act in about 1–2 days. Lactulose has the additional benefit of being effective in the management of hepatic encephalopathy. Sorbitol and mannitol are cheaper and just as effective for laxation. When these sugars are broken down by GI bacteria, they often cause bloating and flatulence.

Box 6.1 Constipation Algorithm

Step 1: Rule out bowel obstruction. (If present, manage symptoms and treat accordingly.)

Step 2: Assess medication regimen for agents that contribute to constipation. *All patients on opioids should receive scheduled laxatives.*

Step 3: Perform a rectal exam. If fecal impaction is present, administer enema or perform manual disimpaction, if appropriate, prior to starting oral laxatives.

Step 4: Give an osmotic laxative.

- **LACTULOSE**

  Route: PO

  Adult Dose: 10–40 g (15–60 mL) every day in divided doses

  Pediatric Dose: 0.7–2 g/kg/day (1–3 mL/kg/day) in divided doses

  Note: Can be given as enema. Mix with water or normal saline (NS) and use rectal balloon catheter. Retain for 30–60 minutes

      or

- **POLYETHYLENE GLYCOL-3350 (PEG-3350)**

  Route: PO

  Adult Dose: 17 g (prepacked packet or ~1 heaping tablespoon—many commercially available bottles have marked caps) dissolved in ~200 mL of fluid (water, milk, juice, soda, broth, tea, coffee, etc.) daily, may increase up to qid

  Pediatric Dose: 0.2–0.8 g/kg/day up to 17 g/day; mix in 100–200 mL of fluid

  Note: Dosing should be adjusted to the desired effect. Infants and young children may require higher doses than those for school-aged children.

Step 5: Add or simultaneously give a stimulant laxative.

- **SENNA**

  Route: PO

  Adult Dose: 8.6 mg tab, start 2 tabs daily, titrate to 2 tabs qid

  Pediatric Dose: 1 month–2 years: 2.2–4.4 mg qhs; 2–6 years: 4.4–6.6 mg qhs; 6–11 years: 8.8–13.2 mg qhs; ≥12 years: 17.6–26.4 mg qhs

      or

- **BISACODYL**

  Route: PO/PR

  Adult Dose:

      PO: 5 mg daily to 15 mg bid

      PR: 10 mg PR daily

  Pediatric Dose:

      PO: 3–12 years: 0.3 mg/kg q24h or 5–10 mg/day; ≥12 years: 5–15 mg/day

      PR: <2 years: 5 mg/day; 2–11 years: 5–10 mg/day; ≥12 years: 10 mg/day

  Note: Only giving stimulant laxatives without an osmotic agent to constipated patients with hardened stool can be very painful and ineffective.

bid, twice daily; PO, oral; PR, rectal; qhs, every bedtime; qid, 4 times daily; SC, subcutaneous.
Sources: Lactulose[6] and Polyethylene glycol 3350.[7]

Electrolyte- and saline-based laxatives are typically sodium- and magnesium-based agents (e.g., sodium phosphate, magnesium citrate). They increase secretion and motility and work on the entire gut, including the small intestines. They act quickly, usually within 30 minutes to 2 hours. These are not good agents if patients require regular maintenance laxatives. One must watch for possible electrolyte imbalance, especially in patients with renal problems.

Lubricant laxatives, such as mineral oil and glycerin suppositories, lubricate the stool surface and decrease water absorption. They act slowly in about 1–3 days and are only appropriate for short-term use.

Enemas create a mechanical flushing and lubricating effect. The instilled volume triggers a mechano-stretch receptor response. The addition of pharmacological content may provide an added stimulant or osmotic effect. Enemas should be used with caution in patients at risk for bleeding, such as those with thrombocytopenia.

For opioid-induced constipation, depending on availability, opioid receptor antagonists, such as naloxone, given orally 0.8 mg PO bid to start, may play a role if patients are not responding to traditional laxatives.

Nausea and Vomiting

Overview

Vomiting or emesis is the forceful emptying of GI contents through one's mouth and can be objectively quantified and characterized, whereas nausea is a subjective sensation of the desire to vomit. Nausea and vomiting are often accompanying symptoms, but patients may experience one without the other. It is important to distinguish between nausea and vomiting and to evaluate each separately. Persistent nausea can cause significant distress, discomfort, and decline, even in the absence of vomiting.

Common causes include the following:
- Dysmotility of the upper GI tract
  - Gastroparesis
- Medications and treatment-related side effects
  - Chemotherapy- and radiotherapy-induced nausea and vomiting (CINV/RINV), digoxin, antibiotics, opioids
- Metabolic disturbances
  - Renal failure (uremia), liver failure, electrolyte imbalances
- Obstruction of GI tract (intrinsic vs. extrinsic)
  - Tumors (both intra -and extraluminal), constipation, ascites
- Infectious etiology
- Vestibular disturbance
- Anxiety
  - Often with an anticipatory component
- Severe pain
- Increased intracranial pressure
  - Tumors, hemorrhage

Box 6.2 Nausea and Vomiting Algorithm

Step 1: Evaluate and treat underlying causes.

Step 2: Select initial therapy based on mostly likely cause of nausea and vomiting. Consider the acronym VOMIT for common causes of nausea/vomiting in palliative care.[8]

Step 2a: Vestibular stimulation

- **HYOSCINE HYDROBROMIDE/SCOPOLAMINE** (anticholinergic)

  Route: PO/PR/IV/SC/TD

  Adult Dose:

  PO: 300 mg tab tid

  SC/IV: 0.3–0.6 mg tid

  TD: 1 mg patch behind the ear every 3 days (4–12 hours initially to take effect)

  Pediatric Dose:

  PO: 150 mg (1/2 tablet) q6h PRN for children over 10 years of age

  SC/IV: 6 mcg/kg/dose (max 0.3 mg/dose) q6–8h PRN

- **DIPHENHYDRAMINE** (H_1 antagonist, mild anticholinergic)

  Route: PO/PR/IV

  Adult Dose: 25–50 mg q4–6h

  Pediatric Dose (>2 years): 0.5–1 mg/kg/dose q4–6h

  Note: May cause paradoxical excitation reaction, especially in children

      or

- **PROMETHAZINE** (H_1 antagonist, mild anticholinergic)

  Route: PO/PR/IM/IV

  Adult Dose: 12.5–25 mg q4–6h PRN

  Pediatric Dose (>2 years): 0.25–1 mg/kg/dose q4–6h PRN; max dose: 25 mg/dose

  Note: May cause paradoxical excitation reaction, especially in children

Step 2b: Obstruction of lower GI tract

- **SENNA** or **BISACODYL** (myenteric plexus neurostimulant)
- **OSMOTIC LAXATIVES**

  See Box 6.1.

Step 2c: Motility problems of upper GI tract

- **METOCLOPRAMIDE** ($5HT_4$ agonist/procholinergic, D_2 antagonist)

  Route: PO/PR/IV/SC

  Route: PO/PR/IV/SC

  Adult Dose: 5–20 mg q6h before meals

  Pediatric Dose: 0.1–0.2 mg/kg/dose (max 10 mg/dose) q6h before meals

  Note: Concurrent use of anticholinergic agents such as hyoscine will blunt or negate the promotility effect of metoclopramide.

  Contraindication: complete bowel obstruction

- **ERYTHROMYCIN** (pro-motilin agent)

  Route: PO/IV

  Adult Dose:
    - PO: 250–500 mg tid before meals
    - IV: 3 mg/kg over 45 minutes q8h

  Pediatric Dose:
    - PO: 3 mg/kg/dose 4 times daily; max increase to 10 mg/kg/dose or 250 mg/dose
    - Note: Not as effective in children over 4 years old

  Note: Tachyphylaxis is common.

Step 2d: Inflammation and edema

- **DEXAMETHASONE** (corticosteroid)

  Route: PO/PR/IV/SC

  Adult Dose: 2–4 mg q8–12h

  Pediatric Dose: 0.15 mg/kg/dose q8–12h

  Note: Also helpful for space-occupying lesions of the brain

- Also consider antihistaminic and anticholinergic agents such as promethazine.

Step 2e: Toxin-stimulating CTZ

- **ONDANSETRON (**$5HT_3$ antagonist)

  Route: PO/PR/IV/SC

  Adult Dose: 4–8 mg q6–8h

  Pediatric Dose (>1 month): 0.1–0.15 mg/kg/dose (max 4–8 mg/dose)

- **HALOPERIDOL** (potent D_2 antagonist)

  Route: PO/PR/IV/SC

  Adult Dose: 0.5–1 mg q4–6h

  Pediatric Dose (>3 years): 0.01–0.1 mg/kg q8h

  also consider

- **PROCHLORPERAZINE (**D_2 antagonist; weak anticholinergic/antihistaminic)

  Route: PO/PR/IV/IM

  Adult Dose:
    - PO: 5–10 mg tid–qid
    - PR: 25 mg bid or 5–10 mg tid–qid
    - IV/IM: 5–10 mg q3–4h up to 40 mg/day

  Pediatric Dose:
    - PO: Children ≥2 years weighing ≥9 kg:

      9–13 kg: 2.5 mg q12–24h as needed; max daily dose: 7.5 mg/day

      >13–18 kg: 2.5 mg q8–12h as needed; max daily dose: 10 mg/day

      >18–39 kg: 2.5 mg q8h or 5 mg q12h as needed; max daily dose: 15 mg/day

      >39 kg: 5–10 mg q6–8h; usual max daily dose: 40 mg/day

- IM: rochlorperazine mesylate: Children ≥2 years weighing ≥9 kg:0.14 mg/kg/dose; 1 dose is usually sufficient; when further doses are needed, convert to oral therapy at equivalent or higher dose
- IV: 0.1–0.15 mg/kg/dose q3–4h; max dose: 10 mg/dose; max daily dose: 40 mg/day (slow IVP <5 mg/min)

Step 3: Special considerations

Step 3a: Malignant bowel obstruction

- **OCTREOTIDE** (somatostatin analog)

  Route: IV/SC

  Adult Dose: 100–400 mcg q8h SC or as a continuous IV infusion

  Pediatric Dose: 1–10 mcg/kg/day SC/IV divided into 1–3 doses a day, or as a continuous IV infusion. Max dose 500 mcg/dose or 1500 mcg/day

  Efficacy is controversial.

Step 3b: Anticipatory nausea/vomiting with an anxiety component

- **LORAZEPAM** (GABA agonist)

  Route: PO/PR/IV/IM

  Adult Dose: 0.5–2 mg q6h

  Pediatric Dose: 0.02–0.05 mg/kg/dose q6h

          or

- **DIAZEPAM**
- Route: PO/PR/IV/SC

  Adult Dose: 2–10 mg bid–qid PRN

          or

- **MIDAZOLAM**
- Route: PO/PR/IV/SC/nasal

  Adult Dose:
  - PO/IV/SC: 1–3 mg q3h PRN
  - Nasal: 5–10 mg intranasal atomizer (may use IV formulation)

  Pediatric Dose:
  - PO/PR: 0.25–0.5 mg/kg q4h PRN
  - Nasal: 0.2 mg/kg q4h PRN

Step 3c: Broad-spectrum approach

- **CHLORPROMAZINE** (primarily antidopaminergic, also provides histaminic, cholinergic, serotonergic, adrenergic blockage)

  Route: PO/IM

  Adult Dose:
  - PO: 10–25 mg q4–6h PRN
  - IM: 12.5–25 mg (up to 50 mg) q3–4h PRN

  Pediatric Dose:
  - Infants ≥6 months, children weighing ≤45.5 kg: PO/IM/IV: 0.55 mg/kg/dose q6–8h as needed; in severe cases, higher doses may be needed

Usual max daily dose: IM/IV:

- Children <5 years or weighing <22.7 kg: 40 mg/day
- Children ≥5 years and adolescents or weighing 22.7 to 45.5 kg: 75 mg/day
- Adolescents weighing >45.5 kg:

Oral: 10–25 mg q4–6h as needed

IM/IV: Initial: 25 mg; if tolerated (no hypotension), then may give 25–50 mg q4–6h as needed

Note: Can be very sedating

Step 4: Assess response. If symptoms persist, increase dose or add agent from different pharmacological class. Consider treatment of concurrent symptoms when present.

- **HALOPERIDOL**: agitation, delirium
- **LORAZEPAM**: anxiety, agitation
- **DIPHENHYDRAMINE**: pruritus, sleeping difficulty
- **DEXAMETHASONE**: disease-related fatigue, anorexia

$5HT_3$, 5-hydroxytriptamine receptor; bid, twice daily; CTZ, chemoreceptor trigger zone; D_2, dopamine receptor; GABA, gamma-amino butyric acid; GI, gastrointestinal; H_1, histamine receptor; IM, intramuscular; IV, intravenous; IVP, intravenous push; PO, oral; PR, rectal; PRN, as needed; qid, 4 times daily; SC, subcutaneous; TD, transdermal; tid, 3 times daily
Sources: Hallenbeck,[8] Chlorpromazine,[9] Diazepam,[10] Erythromycin,[11] Midazolam,[12] Prochlorperazine,[13] and Promethazine.[14]

Management

Because nausea and vomiting are mediated by multiple receptors, it is helpful to match the underlying process to the most effective treatment.[3] One should discontinue or rotate inciting medications whenever possible and avoid or minimize noxious triggers. Adequate hydration and supportive care are essential. Relaxation, distraction techniques, and mindfulness practices can be helpful. Consider treating with stenting, paracentesis, or other interventions and procedures, if appropriate, to address underlying problems.

Pharmacological Management

Following are guidelines for pharmacological management of nausea and vomiting of various etiologies (see Chapter 13 and Box 6.2 for dosing guidelines). Patients often require nonoral routes for medication administration and need continued infusion for optimal symptom management. Many of the medications discussed here can be given subcutaneously and do not require oral or intravenous administration. Note that antidopaminergic agents may cause or exacerbate extrapyramidal symptoms, such as those in patients with Parkinson's disease. Consider complementary medications that work on multiple receptors and on different parts of the nausea–vomiting pathway. However, do not combine treatments that work against each other, such as metoclopramide with promethazine (procholinergic/promotility with anticholinergic agents).

- Vestibular involvement
  - Mediated by cholinergic and histaminic receptors; this is most often associated with motion sickness and dizziness.

- Anticholinergic and antihistaminic medications that cross the blood–brain barrier, penetrating the central nervous system (CNS), work best but tend to be more sedating.
- Medications in this group include hyoscine hydrobromide (scopolamine), promethazine, and diphenhydramine
- Chemoreceptor trigger zone (CTZ)
  - Mediated by dopamine, $5HT_3$ (serotonin), and histamine receptors, the CTZ, located at the base of the fourth ventricle, detects and is especially sensitive to changing levels of toxins in the bloodstream, such as with chemotherapy.
  - Medications in this group include ondansetron (or other available medications in the -setron family that exert $5HT_3$ blockade), prochlorperazine (D_2 dopamine and H_1 histamine blockade), and haloperidol (D_2 blockade).
- Gastroparesis
  - Gastroparesis can be treated with a prokinetic agent via $5HT_4$ agonism and procholinergic activity, such as metoclopramide (also provides D_2 blockade). Erythromycin can be helpful, but tachyphylaxis is common.
- GI obstruction
  - If inflammation and edema are part of the etiology, then steroids like dexamethasone or prednisone may be useful anti-inflammatories (consider a 5-day burst course).
  - Prokinetic neurostimulation medications such as senna and bisacodyl may be considered for lower GI involvement. (Please see above section on constipation.)
- Anxiety or anticipatory nausea/vomiting
  - Benzodiazepines are not good stand-alone antiemetic agents and may increase risk of aspiration, but they are excellent anxiolytic medications in patients for whom this is an issue.
- CNS irritation and space-occupying lesion
  - Initiate steroids if inflammation and edema are present.
- Chlorpromazine (Thorazine)
  - This is an older medication but has a broad spectrum of action that is primarily antidopaminergic, with histamine, cholinergic, and serotonin receptor blockade as well.
- (See section on malignant bowel obstruction for further discussion.)

Malignant Bowel Obstruction (MBO)

Overview

MBO may occur as a result of tumor growing from the GI tract itself or from extrinsic compression due to tumor growing outside the GI tract. Most patients autoconvert between varying degrees of partial to complete obstruction as the GI tract moves within the abdominal cavity. Unresolved complete bowel obstruction without a surgical option will often lead to perforation and is fatal within hours to days. Ongoing MBO causes significant and burdensome symptoms related to the swings between hyperactivity of the gut (hypersecretion and hypermotility) resulting in cramps, nausea, and vomiting, and hypoactivity resulting in gastroparesis, GI stasis, and bloating. The goal of treatment is ongoing support.[4]

Management

Stenting or surgery should be considered, if needed. Decompression via a nasogastric tube or venting gastrostomy can provide some relief but causes discomfort and introduces additional morbidity. IV fluid support should be provided as tolerated for comfort. Management and support of MBO often include monitoring and repletion of electrolytes. Managing symptoms of nausea and vomiting is an essential part of supportive care for MBO. (See section on nausea and vomiting and Chapter 4 on pain management for further discussion.)

Pharmacological Management

Following are guidelines for pharmacological management of MBO (see Chapter 13 for dosing guidelines.)

Octreotide, a somatostatin analog, decreases secretions and decreases motility while allowing the GI tract to maintain reabsorption and other key functions. Its efficacy in MBO is controversial, but for refractory patients it is often trialed when available. It can be given subcutaneously as an injection or as a continuous infusion. Patients may need a few days to see the full effect of this medication. Steroids, like dexamethasone, may often be helpful to decrease inflammation. Promotility agents, such as metoclopramide, may be used in partial bowel obstruction but should be avoided in complete or severe obstruction. These medications may be used in conjunction with each other and provide a synergistic effect.

Anticholinergics, especially those that do not cross the blood–brain barrier (e.g., glycopyrrolate or hyoscine butylbromide), may help decrease GI secretion and motility and thus provide bowel rest. A proton pump inhibitor and H_2 blocker may be used to decrease gastric secretion. For patients with complete obstruction or bowel perforation and are not surgical candidates, aggressive symptom management with opioids for pain is essential. Sedation is often a desirable side effect for these patients, and one should choose anticholinergic agents that readily cross the blood–brain barrier, such as hyoscine hydrobromide (scopolamine).

Anorexia and Cachexia

Overview

Anorexia is the loss of appetite for food—patients lack the sensation of hunger; it is often an associated symptom in patients with GI symptoms discussed in this chapter. Cachexia is a wasting syndrome of weight loss and muscle atrophy, often characterized by weakness and fatigue.[5] With treatment and reversal of the underlying disease process, whenever possible, appetite should return. However, the end stage of many conditions (e.g., cancer, HIV/AIDS) and in actively dying patients anorexia, cachexia, or both are often part of the dying process.

Anorexia must be distinguished from starvation, where hunger is present and patients are being *deprived* of adequate food intake. Starvation, along with malnutrition, is commonly encountered in humanitarian crises.

Management

It is paramount to provide education and supportive counseling and to address psychosocial and cultural concerns associated with anorexia and cachexia. The eating and sharing of meals is a deeply ingrained human activity that is transcultural. It is often very distressing for family members to witness the process of anorexia and cachexia. Smaller portions and eating for pleasure can be satisfying for many patients. Finding alternate ways of feeding whenever possible may be important for patients, family members, and caregivers. However, clinically, artificial enteral or parenteral nutrition offers no benefit in terminal and end-stage conditions. In end-of-life care, finding alternate ways besides feeding for family members and caregivers to nurture and care for the patient who is anorexic and cachectic is important. Well intended but forced feeding may lead to distress and suffering such as pain, nausea, and vomiting, without the intended benefits. Eating when desired should be for pleasure, adequate caloric/nutritional intake is neither a priority nor a goal in management.

Pharmacological Management

Following are guidelines for pharmacological management of anorexia and cachexia (see Chapter 13 for dosing guidelines).

Treatment of reversible conditions (e.g., oral thrush, constipation) and optimal management of chronic conditions are paramount. Early satiety may be seen in patients with compression of the stomach from ascites, hepatomegaly, or other forms of outlet obstruction and gastroparesis. Metoclopramide, a promotility agent, can be used if the patient has symptoms of early satiety and delayed gastric emptying.

Certain medications have an orexigenic (appetite-stimulating) effect but do not reverse the underlying pathology and do not address the issue of cachexia. However, for the purposes of palliation, glucocorticoid steroids such as dexamethasone can be helpful. Antidepressive and antipsychotic agents such as mirtazapine and olanzapine, when available, may be selected for their profile of desirable side effects, such as appetite stimulation and weight gain. Progestin agents such as megestrol are not usually recommended because of the cost and prothrombotic profile, which is especially problematic for many cancer patients.

References

1. Watson M, Lucas C, Hoy A, Back I, eds. Diarrhoea. In: *Oxford Handbook of Palliative Care*. Oxford, UK: Oxford University Press; 2006:258–261.

2. Bruera E, Fadul N. Constipation and diarrhea. In: Bruera E, Higginson I, Ripamonti C, von Gunten C, eds. *Textbook of Palliative Medicine*. London: Hodder Arnold; 2006:554–567.

3. Wood G, Shega J, Lynch B, Von Roenn J. Management of intractable nausea and vomiting in patients at the end of life. *JAMA*. 2007;298(10):1196–1207.

4. Ripamonti C. Bowel obstruction. In: Bruera E, Higginson I, Ripamonti C, von Gunten C, eds. *Textbook of Palliative Medicine*. London: Hodder Arnold; 2006:588-600.

5. Watson M, Lucas C, Hoy A, Back I, eds. Anorexia. In: *Oxford Handbook of Palliative Care*: Oxford, UK: Oxford University Press; 2006:266–267.

6. Lactulose. Lexicomp, *UpToDate*. https://www.uptodate.com. Accessed March 29, 2019.

7. Polyethylene glycol 3350. Lexicomp, *UpToDate*. https://www.uptodate.com. Accessed March 29, 2019.

8. Hallenbeck JL. Non-pain symptom management. In: *Palliative Care Perspectives*. New York: Oxford University Press; 2003.

9. Chlorpromazine. Lexicomp. *UpToDate*. https://www.uptodate.com. Accessed March 30, 2019.

10. Diazepam. Lexicomp. *UpToDate*. https://www.uptodate.com. Accessed March 30, 2019.

11. Erythromycin. Lexicomp. *UpToDate*. https://www.uptodate.com. Accessed March 30, 2019.

12. Midazolam. Lexicomp. *UpToDate*. https://www.uptodate.com. Accessed March 30, 2019.

13. Prochlorperazine. Lexicomp. *UpToDate*. https://www.uptodate.com. Accessed March 30, 2019.

14. Promethazine. Lexicomp. *UpToDate*. https://www.uptodate.com. Accessed March 30, 2019.

Chapter 7

Delirium and Acute Anxiety

Kevin Bezanson and Stephanie Rogers

Introduction

While reactions to stressors faced in humanitarian crises take many forms, often they present with acute confusion and agitation. Those individuals with life-threatening or palliative illnesses, whether pre-existing or as a result of the crisis, are especially vulnerable. This chapter reviews the assessment of these patients, first to identify and treat those with delirium, in the attempt to reverse it and optimally manage associated symptoms. Second, the management of acute anxiety and agitation of a primarily psychological origin is addressed (see also Chapter 16).

Delirium

Background

Delirium is an acute confusional state precipitated by a medical illness or injury that is its primary underlying cause. It is very common in patients with life-limiting illnesses.[1] It is often very distressing for patients and caregivers because it interferes with the ability the ability to meaningfully interact, assess, and treat patients in every aspect of their care. Prevention and early identification through addressing potentially reversible causes, careful prescribing and de-prescribing of medications, and behavioral interventions are vital to maximizing potential resolution (see Table 7.1). Delirium is more likely to be reversible earlier in illness/injury trajectory, and much less near end of life, requiring discretion in utilization of appropriate and available investigations or treatments. It is also important to engage patients and families, as their interpretations of causes and appropriate treatments from a spiritual and/or cultural perspective may differ significantly from the biomedical perspective.

Diagnosis

Distinguishing delirium from other causes of confusion is sometimes challenging, but a critical first step to appropriate management. The Confusion Assessment Method[2,3] is a practical tool using four cardinal features to help identify and distinguish delirium from other causes:

A. Acute onset and fluctuating course
   • Change from patient's baseline developing over hours to days
   • Symptoms and severity vary over the course of the day

B. Inattention
- Difficulty maintaining focus or concentration in conversation or activities

C. Disorganized thinking
- Inappropriate, confusing, illogical, or tangential responses

D. Altered level of consciousness
- Can be hyper-alert and vigilant, or drowsy and lethargic

The presence of both A **and** B along with C **and/or** D strongly supports the diagnosis.

Table 7.1. PCHC Delirium Algorithm

Step 1: Diagnose delirium on the basis of clinical symptoms (acute onset and fluctuating course, inattention, disorganized thinking, altered level of consciousness).

Step 2: Identify and treat potential causes (medications, infections, shock, trauma, intoxication or withdrawal, electrolyte abnormalities, neurological, elimination).

Step 3: Implement behavioral/nonpharmacological interventions.
- Enlist support of family/caregivers to provide support and supervision for safety.
- Maintain daytime routines and nighttime routines to support orientation and sleep.
- Assist with nutrition and hydration.
- Ensure sensory deficits are addressed as much as possible to enhance communication.
- Avoid tethering medical devices and restraints.

Step 4: Use neuroleptic agents **only if safety concerns** are not addressed by other measures.
- Use the lowest dose possible, assessing for adverse effects, and discontinuing as soon as able.

- **HALOPERIDOL** (first-line agent)

Route: PO/SL/IV

Adult Dose: 0.5–1 mg q4–6h

Pediatric Dose (>3 years, injection >18 years): 0.01–0.1 mg/kg q8h

- **CHLORPROMAZINE** (second-line agent, **only if sedation required for safety**)

Route: PO/IV

Adult Dose: 10 mg PO q4–6h, 25 mg PR q6–12h, 5–10 mg IM/IV q8–12 h

Pediatric Dose: 0.1 mg/kg/dose PO/PR q6–8h, 0.1–0.15 mg/kg/dose IM/IV q8–12h

Step 5: Consider use of benzodiazepines **only if safety concerns persist despite previous measures** (exception: alcohol withdrawal).
- May exacerbate agitation, monitor closely for response.

- **LORAZEPAM**

Route: PO/SL/PR/IV/SC

Adult Dose: 0.5–2 mg q6h

Pediatric Dose: 0.02–0.05 mg/kg/dose q6h

- **DIAZEPAM**

Route: PO/IV/PR/SC

Adult Dose: 2.5–10 mg q6h PRN

Pediatric Dose: 0.05–0.3mg/kg q6h PRN

IM, intramuscular; IV, intravenous; PO, oral; PR, rectal; PRN, as needed; SC, subcutaneous; SL, sublingual.

Other features commonly found include the following:

- Perceptual disturbances such as hallucinations and delusions
- Disturbance in sleep/wake cycle
- Disorientation to person, place, or time
- Memory impairment especially for recent events
- Psychomotor agitation or retardation

The *Diagnostic and Statistical Manual of Mental Disorders,* 5th ed. (DSM-5)[4] emphasizes that there should be evidence that the cognitive changes have been precipitated by a medical condition, rather than a primary cognitive/psychiatric condition (e.g., dementia, depression, schizophrenia). However, delirium can present as an acute worsening of baseline symptoms in patients with these conditions, making diagnosis more challenging.

Another clinically relevant diagnostic distinction is that delirium has three subtypes[5] that alter its presentation significantly. The hyperactive type is much more likely to come to attention because of accompanying agitation, but the hypoactive type is perhaps more common and easily missed because patients are more quietly confused. The mixed type recognizes that both can coexist in the same patient due to the fluctuating course of the illness, sometimes causing diagnostic difficulty.

Management

Delirium management requires a multifaceted approach in what is often a very stressful situation for patients, families, and care providers. It is necessary to simultaneously identify and treat underlying causes, while managing associated distressing symptoms, and supporting the patient and family.[6] Enlisting family/caregivers to the extent possible in care is essential at every step, especially in humanitarian crisis settings where these patients needs are high and resources are limited.

Identify and Treat Underlying Causes

This requires adaptation to the available resources for investigations and treatment of potential causes, particularly given the constrained realities often present humanitarian crises. It also requires judgment based on the likelihood of reversibility, recalling that patients nearer to end of life are less likely to have a reversible cause identified. In circumstances where the cause is identified and irreversible, or it is not possible to identify or treat the cause(s), a focus on comfort measures should take precedence.

In most cases there are multiple causes contributing to the delirium many of which overlap and intersect.[7] In humanitarian crises, some of the key causes to assess for in history and examination, relevant potential investigations, and basic management are outlined below. Access to these investigations and treatments may vary widely in humanitarian settings.

Medications

Precipitating medications include the following:

- Anticholinergics—antispasmodics, antihistamines, antinauseants, neuroleptics/antipsychotics
- Sedatives—benzodiazepines, other sleep aids

- Pain medications—opiates, muscle relaxants, tricyclic antidepressants, anticonvulsants
- Other—steroids, antimalarials, traditional medicines

Discontinue or taper any medications that are not needed using the lowest doses possible.

Infections

- Malaria, encephalitis, meningitis, pneumonia, wound infection, sepsis, cholera, typhoid fever, syphilis
- Laboratory tests and cultures
- Antimicrobials and other measures to treat infection

Dehydration/Shock

- Laboratory tests and assess for underlying cause
- Intravenous fluids and/or oral rehydration, blood transfusion

Musculoskeletal/Organ Trauma

- Laboratory tests and diagnostic imaging
- Stabilization of injuries and surgery

Intoxication/Withdrawal/Overdose

- Alcohol, opiates, etc.
- Laboratory tests
- Supportive measures (e.g., thiamine), reversal (e.g., naloxone)

Electrolyte Abnormalities

- Hypercalcemia, hyponatremia, hypoglycemia
- Laboratory tests
- Correction intravenously/orally, dialysis

Neurological

- Trauma, cerebrovascular, brain metastases
- Diagnostic Imaging
- Anti-inflammatories, anticoagulants, surgery

Elimination

- Urinary retention, constipation, obstruction
- Catheterization, laxatives/disimpaction, nasogastric tube

Behavioral (Nonpharmacological) Interventions

Behavioral interventions are often readily available in humanitarian settings, and can be undertaken by family and other nonclinical providers. However, some reassurance and guidance may be needed to enlist effective participation. Explaining the possible causes and management plan identified by healthcare providers, listening to family or other caregivers thoughts about behaviors of concern and other contributing factors, and giving specific instructions for support are essential to caring for a delirious patient.

The normal day/night cycle is often compromised or reversed in delirium. Strategies to maintain it help minimize symptom burden. Encouraging mental stimulation during the day by access to light, conversations and reminiscing, games, physical engagement, and avoiding naps are helpful. Specifically whenever possible being out of bed and in a chair, and out of a room or shelter are key. Maintaining mealtimes and supporting hydration and nutrition through feeding assistance help with reorientation and treat potential contributing factors. Nighttime is equally important, especially supporting restful sleep as much as possible. This includes a darkened room, minimizing environmental noise (including eye shades and ear plugs if available), and avoiding waking for care unless absolutely needed.

Other important practical measures include using sensory aids when available (e.g., glasses, hearing aids, dentures) to enhance communication and orientation. Even small familiar items from home can provide reassurance, recognizing these are often unavailable in humanitarian emergencies. Avoid if all possible tethering medical devices such as intravenous lines that can compromise safety and increase agitation.

Taken together behavioral interventions are effective[8] and should be the mainstay of supportive management of delirium in palliative patients.

Physical Restraints and Pharmacological Management

Physical restraints should only be considered in cases where physical safety is at risk, and other measures have failed. If needed they should be minimized and reassessed regularly as they can prolong the delirium.

Though widely used, current evidence does not support the routine use of neuroleptic/antipsychotic medications for prevention or treatment of delirium.[9] Evidence particularly in palliative populations is limited, and largely based on consensus expert opinion.[10] Recent studies have questioned their effectiveness and raised concerns about harms.[11] They should be reserved for cases where a delirious patient poses a safety risk to themselves, caregivers, or staff. Other behavioral (see previous section on behavioral interventions) and treatment measures (see previous section on identifying and treating underlying causes) should be provided to full extent possible.

With these caveats, the mainstay of pharmacologic treatment of agitated delirium is the neuroleptic/antipsychotic haloperidol (see Chapter 13). It should be used in the lowest dose and frequency needed to control symptoms, patients monitored for adverse effects especially extrapyramidal symptoms, and discontinued as soon as possible.[8,12] The other neuroleptic that could be considered if haloperidol is ineffective and sedation is required for safety is chlorpromazine (see Chapter 13) using the same minimal use principles.

The other class of medications sometimes used to treat severe agitated delirium is benzodiazepines, but should be reserved only for cases when extreme sedation is needed. Generally these medications are avoided in delirium due to lack of evidence of benefit, risks of adverse events, and concerns about worsening delirium, except in cases of alcohol withdrawal,[13] While two recent randomized controlled trials have raised questions about a potential role,[11,14] benzodiazepines would generally be reserved for refractory cases where sedation is the desired outcome using either lorazepam or diazepam (see Chapter 13).

Acute Anxiety

Overview

Anxiety and agitation are very common and normal responses to traumatic events experienced in acute humanitarian crises and emergencies, but can still result in severe symptoms and distress. They are normally time-limited, and as such they can be usually be managed with supportive measures alone. In more severe cases, medications can be used on a temporary, short-term basis to target specific symptoms. It is also important to acknowledge patients and families may interpret the cause, and appropriate treatment, from a more spiritual and/or cultural perspective, rather than a purely psychological and/or medical one.

Diagnosis

Often presentations are a combination of emotional, psychological, and physical symptoms.[15,16] Emotions of fear, panic, sadness, despair, behaviors of screaming, crying, withdrawal, aggression, and symptoms of disorientation, shortness of breath, heart palpitations, nausea and vomiting, sweating, chills, prostration, and pseudo-seizures may occur. These tend to occur in episodes of limited duration, with periods of near normalcy in between, helping distinguish from delirium. However, if these episodes become more frequent and pervasive, they can indicate potentially more severe mental health conditions such as post-traumatic stress disorder, depression, and anxiety disorders requiring more intensive management (see Chapter 16).

Management

Behavioral and Psychosocial (Nonpharmacological) Interventions

This is the mainstay of treatment, and first recourse in addressing anxiety, encompassed in the principles of psychological first aid.[17] It is important during an episode to provide a safe physical space to the extent possible. Providing reassurance and support, and nonjudgmental listening may be of great value. Patients need to be educated that their reactions are normal given the trauma they have encountered, and usually reduce with time. It is important to recognize the key role of family and other community supports, and with guidance and permission from the patient, seek to strengthen those connections. Other practical needs should be addressed to the extent possible to enhance a sense of safety and security. It may also be helpful to recommend relaxation techniques such as breathing exercises, distraction, physical activity, prayer, and traditional practices.

Pharmacological Treatments

These should be limited to short-term, time-limited (usually <1 week) measures to treat severe and persistent insomnia or panic symptoms not responding to behavioral and psychosocial interventions.[15] Typically lorazepam or diazepam can be used in the lowest effective dose (see Chapter 13). Amitriptyline can also be used for sleep, and has the advantage that it can be used longer term more safely, and for treatment of anxiety disorders and depression.

References

1. Hosie A, Davidson PM, Agar M, Sanderson CR, Phillips J. Delirium prevalence, incidence, and implications for screening in specialist palliative care inpatient settings: a systematic review. *Palliat Med.* 2013;27(6):486–498.

2. Inouye, S, van Dyck, C, Alessi, C, et al. Clarifying confusion: the Confusion Assessment Method. *Ann Int Med.* 1990;113(12); 941–948.

3. Wei LA, Fearing MA, Sternberg EJ, Inouye, SK. The Confusion Assessment Method (CAM): a systematic review of current usage. *J Am Geriatr Soc.* 2008;56(5):823–830.

4. American Psychiatric Association. *Diagnostic and Statistical Manual of Mental Disorders.* 5th ed. Washington DC: 2013.

5. Meagher D. Motor subtypes of delirium. *Int Rev Psychiatry.* 2009;21(1):59–73.

6. Chapter 7 Delirium. In: *The Pallium Palliative Pocketbook: A Peer-Reviewed, Referenced Resource.* 2nd ed. Ottawa: Pallium Canada; 2016:172–185.

7. Lawlor PG, Gagnon B, Mancini IL, et al. *Arch Intern Med.* 2000;160(6):786–794.

8. Bush SH, Kanji S, Pereira JL, et al. Treating an established episode of delirium in palliative care: expert opinion and review of the current evidence base with recommendations for future development. *J Pain Symptom Manage.* 2014;48(2):231–248.

9. Neufeld KJ, Yue J, Robinson TN, Inouye SK, Needham DM. Antipsychotic medication for prevention and treatment of delirium in hospitalized adults: a systematic review and meta-analysis. *J Am Geriatr Soc.* 2016;64(4):705–714.

10. Bush SH, Bruera E, Lawlor PG, et al. Clinical practice guidelines for delirium management: potential application in palliative care. *J Pain Symptom Manage.* 2014;48(2):249–258.

11. Agar MR, Lawlor PG, Quinn S, et al. Efficacy of oral risperidone, haloperidol, or placebo for symptoms of delirium among patients in palliative care: a randomized clinical trial. *JAMA Intern Med.* 2017;177(1):34–42.

12. Hui D, Dev R, Bruera E. Neuroleptics in the management of delirium in patients with advanced cancer. *Curr Opin Support Palliat Care.* 2016;10(4): 316–323.

13. Lonergan E, Luxenberg J, Areosa Sastre A. Benzodiazepines for delirium. *Cochrane Database of Systematic Reviews* 2009; Issue 4.

14. Hui D, Frisbee-Hume S, Wilson A, Dibaj SS, Nguyen T, De La Cruz, M. Effect of lorazepam with haloperidol vs haloperidol alone on agitated delirium in patients with advanced cancer receiving palliative care: a randomized clinical trial. *JAMA.* 2017; 318(11): 1047–1056.

15. Médecins Sans Frontières. Chapter 11: Mental disorders in adults. In: *Clinical Guidelines—Diagnosis and Treatment Manual.* Médecins Sans Frontières; 2018:307–311. https://medicalguidelines.msf.org/viewport/MG/en/guidelines-16681097.html. Accessed April 4, 2019.

16. World Health Organization and United Nations High Commissioner for Refugees. *mhGAP Humanitarian Intervention Guide (mhGAP-HIG): Clinical Management of Mental, Neurological and Substance Use Conditions in Humanitarian Emergencies.* Geneva: WHO, 2015. https://www.who.int/mental_health/publications/mhgap_hig/en/. Accessed April 4, 2019.

17. World Health Organization, War Trauma Foundation and World Vision International. *Psychological First Aid: Guide for Field Workers.* WHO: Geneva. 2011. https://www.who.int/mental_health/publications/guide_field_workers/en/. Accessed April 4, 2019.

Chapter 8

Skin Conditions in Crisis Areas

Marcia Glass, Carrie Kovarik, Mara Haseltine,
Sandra L. Freiwald, and Susan Barbour

Introduction

Many severely or terminally ill patients in natural disasters, conflict zones, and epidemics experience skin afflictions. A basic understanding of the most common and urgent skin disorders in these settings is essential to providing comprehensive care to affected patients. For example, in the days after the 2004 Asian tsunami, an Indonesian hospital reported 265 skin complaints among 235 patients seeking care.[1] Similarly, a study after the 2015 Nepalese earthquake found that 52.3% of 7,326 patients had direct or indirect dermatoses following the earthquake.[2]

As with any conditions in crisis areas, consideration of the psychological stressors facing patients in these conditions is essential. Psychoemotional stress can aggravate many skin conditions, such as rosacea, psoriasis, eczema, acne, urticaria, seborrheic dermatitis, atopic dermatitis, and alopecia areata. It can also be linked to induction of an intense need to scratch or pick the skin (neurotic excoriation) or pull out the hair (trichotillomania).[1,2]

Exposure-Related Wounds

Tetanus

Many traumatic injuries can put the patient at risk for the development of tetanus, especially in areas where routine vaccinations are uncommon. At-risk wounds include burns, snake bites, gunshot wounds, open fractures, and any other wound with significant contamination and devitalized tissue.

Patients with tetanus-prone wounds whose immunization status is unknown should be given 250–500 units human tetanus immunoglobulin. They should also receive a dose of Td (tetanus toxoid and diphtheria toxoid) intramuscularly and complete the immunization series. This includes 3 doses (0.5 mL IM) of Td. The second dose is given in 4–8 weeks and the third is given 6–12 months after the second.

Burns

Burns can be caused by chemicals (including acids, alkali, toxic compounds, and chemical warfare agents), friction, cold, heat, and radiation damage. First-degree burns cause only superficial damage; second-degree, partial-thickness burns affect the epidermis and the dermis; and third-degree burns penetrate the dermis and affect deeper tissues. Severe, third-degree burns can result in devitalization of muscle and even bone and may require surgical intervention. In rare cases, infarction may lead to auto-amputation of affected areas.

For initial treatment for major burns extinguish the flames, which might include rolling the victim if clothing is on fire. Use large amounts of water to dilute an agent causing chemical burns, copiously irrigate affected eyes, keep any phosphorus (from chemical warfare) still in contact with victim's skin covered with water, and supply 5–10 L/min of humidified oxygen if the airway is affected. If the patient is showing signs of shock, the legs can be elevated. If the burns occurred within an enclosed space, be watchful for signs of inhalation injury, including facial burns, hoarseness, stridor, or carbonaceous sputum. If mechanical ventilation is available, such patients should be intubated as soon as possible.

Burns should be irrigated with cool water or saline to remove loose dirt and skin then washed gently with soap and water and dried with a clean towel. Peel or trim loose, necrotic skin, but do not remove any viable-appearing skin. Drain large blisters with a sterile needle near the base of the blister, but do not remove the blister roof. Cover the burn with Vaseline gauze and change every day. Maintain mobility of the wound and avoid dependent positioning. Give oral rehydration solution and/or IV fluids. Place a clean sheet under the patient and cover with another sheet and clean blanket. Only give antibiotics if the wound is showing signs of infection. Ketamine can be used for acute pain control and during subsequent dressing changes.[3,4]

Snake Bites

Snake bites result in a range of skin reactions, with simple fang marks on one extreme and marked extremity swelling, subcutaneous ecchymoses and bullae, and severe systemic symptoms, including coagulopathy and cardiovascular collapse, on the other.

Treatment involves immobilizing the bitten extremity by splinting. Keep the limb padded at heart level. Encourage the victim to drink liquids until IV access is possible. Victims may also need analgesia, transfusions, fluid resuscitation, antibiotics, steroids, and antivenom, as available.[4]

Open Fracture

An open fracture is an injury that includes disruption of the skin and a broken bone. This fracture is by definition contaminated and is prone to the development of sepsis or chronic infection.

If hospital care is not immediately available, treat with a clean dressing, splint, and give broad-spectrum antibiotics. If hospital care is delayed, the wound should be irrigated with water. Angulated or malpositioned fractures should be realigned and placed in traction. Visible bone ends can be rinsed with dilute 10% povidone-iodine solution. Open fractures of the lower leg are at high risk for the development of compartment syndrome, so consultation with a surgical specialist should be sought as soon as possible. [4]

Traumatic Amputation

Treatment involves controlling hemorrhage with direct pressure. A tourniquet should only be used as a life-saving measure as it can lead to further tissue loss.

Without cooling, an amputated part remains viable for 4–6 hours; with cooling, viability can be extended to 18 hours.

Cleanse the amputated part with water, wrap it in a moistened sterile gauze or towel, place it in a plastic bag, and transport on ice or snow, if available. Do not transport in direct contact with ice or ice water. Make sure the amputated part accompanies the victim throughout the evacuation process.[4]

Firearm Trauma

This trauma differs in severity based on the type of weapon and ammunition used.

To treat firearm trauma follow basic trauma resuscitation, immobilization, wound care, and stabilization for transport. Remove the weapon from the area in which you are providing medical care. If a neck wound with an expanding hematoma is present, perform endotracheal intubation. If intubation is not possible, perform cricothyrotomy. Provide needle or chest tube decompression for a tension pneumothorax. Hemothorax should be treated with tube thoracostomy. Evacuated blood can be filtered and retransfused to the patient. Treat a sucking chest wound with Vaseline gauze secured on ¾ sides to allow egress of air from the thorax. Control external bleeding with direct pressure and compression wraps. Treat the patient for shock and hypothermia. Keep affected extremities elevated. Use forceps to remove superficial ballistic fragments. For powder burns, remove as much powder residue as possible. [4]

Anthrax

Anthrax is a zoonosis caused by *Bacillus anthracis* acquired from infected cattle, horses, mules, sheep, and goats. It can also be used as a biological warfare agent. The characteristic sign is a red, blistering edema. The blisters become hemorrhagic and necrotic. They eventually form black crusts and are accompanied by systemic signs.[3]

Treatment is with high doses of penicillin and tetracycline.

High-Risk Wounds

These wounds include animal or human bites to the hand, wrist, or foot, over a major joint, or through the cheek; any cat bite or scratch; deep puncture wounds; deep wounds to the hand or foot; wounds with crushed or devitalized tissue; or wounds older than 8 hours to the extremity, 12 hours to the torso, and 24 hours to the face and scalp. None of these wounds should be closed in the field.

For treatment, after irrigation and debridement, pack the wound open with saline-moistened gauze. Cover the packed wound with a conforming bandage, splint the extremity in an anatomical position and elevate it. Start broad-spectrum antibiotics, such as ampicillin-sulbactam. The wound can be closed secondarily after 4–5 days if no signs of infection develop. [4]

Frostbite

Frostbite ranges in severity based on whether tissue loss occurs. Signs and symptoms include numbness, erythema, edema, blue mottling, insensate skin with diminished pliability, blisters, mummification, and bony involvement.

Preferred field treatment is rapid rewarming (with water warmed to 40° to 42° Celsius) and prevention of refreezing after thaw. Replace constricting and wet clothing with dry, loose garments. Keep victims well hydrated, administer oxygen, elevate the injured extremity, protect them from further trauma, place gauze between the digits to prevent maceration, prohibit tobacco use, do not rupture blisters but do irrigate them, allow active motion, give analgesics including ibuprofen, and use antibiotics for extensive injury or ruptured blisters. [4]

Trench Foot

Trench foot refers to prolonged exposure to nonfreezing cold and wet conditions leading to neurovascular damage without ice crystals. It starts as red skin that becomes pale and swollen. It may lead to diffuse discoloration, mottling, blistering, ulceration, paresthesias, and numbness.

To treat trench foot keep the affected area dry and warm. Initial treatment is similar to that for frostbite, but rewarming is not necessary. [4]

Floodwater Infections

Vibro vulnificans

Vibro vulnificans is a flood-associated disease, most commonly acquired when an open wound is exposed to saltwater. It can cause fulminant cellulitis and myositis. Oral exposure leads to septicemia with watery diarrhea, fever, chills, nausea, vomiting, and abdominal pain. Patients with liver disease, HIV, diabetes, and other forms of immunosuppression are at highest risk.

Treatment involves supportive care and use of doxycycline and ceftazidine. It may require aggressive surgical debridement if a necrotizing soft tissue infection develops.[1]

Aeromonas hydrophila

Aeromonas hydrophila shares environmental attributes with the *Vibrio* species but is primarily found in freshwater. Humans often acquire this infection orally, and it usually presents with gastroenteritis. Immunocompromised patients are most at risk. Infection can present as cellulitis after an open wound is exposed to freshwater. Necrotizing fasciitis or myonecrosis can occur later, with severe pain, swelling, serosanguinous bullae, gas gangrene, and sepsis.

Treatment is with broad-spectrum antibiotics; surgical debridement may be required. [1]

Chromobacterium violaceum

Chromobacterium violaceum is commonly found on decaying organic matter in tropical and subtropical freshwater and soil. Skin disease usually results from minor skin breaks being exposed to contaminated water. Cutaneous manifestations include cellulitis with pustules and nodules or ecthyma gangrenosum-like lesions after dissemination. Initial infection can rapidly progress to fulminant sepsis with multiorgan involvement. Visceral abscesses can rapidly develop.

Treatment involves surgical drainage of cutaneous and visceral abscesses, along with several weeks of broad-spectrum IV antibiotics.[1]

Mucormycosis

Mucormycosis is a fungus that is particularly dangerous in immunocompromised hosts. Skin infections occur after traumatic injury to the skin and exposure to the environment. Cutaneous disease usually presents as refractory infection of a simple abrasion or traumatic wound. If untreated, *Mucor* infection can progress to severe, extensive tissue necrosis, gangrene, and severe or fatal systemic infection.

Treatment is with aggressive surgical debridement, systemic antifungals, particularly amphotericin B.[1]

General Skin Care

Pruritus

This is a symptom in many skin disorders. In refractory pruritus, the patient's skin can become thickened and form a dry, raised plaque with a darkened skin color known as lichenification. Some parasitic infections, such as schistosomiasis, may cause intermittent, itchy wheals or urticaria. If additional members of the household are also itching, and the patient has itchy bumps on the genitals, finger webs, and other areas, scabies should be considered. Other causes of pruritus include iron deficiency, renal failure, thyroid disease, liver disease, lymphoproliferative diseases, drug reactions, and psychological disorders.

Treatment is based on the underlying cause. If no cause can be found, symptomatic relief can be attempted with topical steroids, antihistamines, emulsifying ointments, menthol cream, oatmeal soaks, gabapentin, and amitriptyline, as appropriate. [5–7.]

Edema

Edema is usually caused by the accumulation of fluid in the tissue. The swelling is initially soft but can harden with time from fibrosis or scarring. Edema can also become secondarily infected with bacteria and appear weepy and bumpy. If area is warm and tender, this may suggest an infection.

Filariasis

Filariasis can cause pronounced extremity and genitourinary swelling, with a foul-smelling discharge.

Mycetoma

Mycetoma causes unilateral, painless, and localized swelling, often to the feet, with draining sinus tracts.

Buruli Ulcers

These are mycobacterial infections that cause an indolent, painless ulcer with undermined edges. Before a Buruli ulceration occurs on a limb, the skin surface is usually swollen or may blister. Once a Buruli ulcer forms, there is usually pronounced swelling around the ulcer.

Kaposi's Sarcoma

Kaposi's sarcoma (KS) often causes edema, with overlying purple, red or dark-colored patches, papules, or nodules. Patients often also have lymphadenopathy in the affected limb, and the swelling tends to be asymmetrical.

Heart, Liver, and Kidney

Heart, liver, and kidney failure may cause bilateral leg swelling but is usually relatively symmetrical and accompanied by other systemic symptoms.

Treatment will target the underlying cause. In general, treatment involves massage for lymphedema, compression with elastic bandages and leg elevation, moisturizers to prevent skin breakdown, leg movement through walking or passive movements, and support stockings. Topical steroids and diuretics can be used to improve skin symptoms from noninfectious causes of leg edema. Antibiotics can be used for superimposed infection, along with targeted antiparasitics and antifungals (depending on the cause), and antiretrovirals and/or chemotherapy for KS. [5,7,8]

Fungating Tumors

These tumors frequently cause pain, odor, excessive drainage, and bleeding, which can lead to social isolation and significant distress. It is not unusual to see maggots in the wound if care has not been optimized.

Treatment (for palliation) is as follows:

Pain: Premedicate before dressing. Soak any dressings that are adhered to the tissue to prevent bleeding and pain. Rinse with normal saline or rock salt (2 teaspoons or 10 g) boiled into 1 L warm water.

Odor: Remove loose debris with rinsing. Crush metronidazole tablets into powder and apply to the wound by shaking or throwing the powder onto the wound. Careful debridement of thick, necrotic, loose tissue can be attempted for severe odor. Cover entire tumor with Vaseline gauze or similar non-stick dressing to trap odors. This can also help with hemostasis and clear up anaerobic infection. Metronidazole tablets can also be inserted in a sinus or orifice. This is useful for rectal and cervical cancer.

Drainage: For excessive drainage, use disposable baby diapers to soak up drainage and protect clothing. Secure in place using wide gauze wraps.

Bleeding: Try to minimize bleeding by preventing dressing from sticking to the tumor. For mild to moderate bleeding, apply pressure for 10–15 minutes. For persistent or severe bleeding, consider Tranexamic acid 650 mg (crushed) or 1 g injectable in 5–10 mL saline applied to gauze tid. One can also try 1:1000 adrenaline-soaked gauze or sucralfate 1–2 g/10 mL suspension bid applied to the wound. For terminal hemorrhage, it is best to use dark towels and have a plan in place for sedation and pain relief.

Maggot removal: Use hydrogen peroxide to rinse the wound and pick off the maggots as they come to the surface.

Chronic Skin Conditions

Conditions such as eczema, psoriasis, and bullous pemphigoid can all flare during intensely stressful situations.

Even if patients in crisis areas do not have access to their regular medications for these chronic conditions, symptomatic relief can often be achieved with oral steroids. Ensure that an adequate supply is given to the patient so they can either taper the steroids or continue their current dose.

Superimposed Bacterial Infections

Such infections may occur on damaged skin. Common bacteria causing them include *Streptococcus, Staphylococcus, and Pseudomonas*. Injured skin is more susceptible to bacterial infection, which can present as cellulitis, boils, pustules, furuncles, and necrotizing fasciitis.

Treatment is with broad-spectrum penicillins, surgical debridement as needed, and daily dressings. If you are in an area with a high prevalence of methicillin-resistant *Staphylococcus aureus* (MRSA), treatment regimens may need to be modified. Dilute vinegar and bleach (diluted to barely smell like a swimming pool) washings can also be used. Necrotizing soft tissue infections requires urgent surgical debridement.

Malnutrition

Malnutrition can cause a variety of skin manifestations and may require specialized intervention. For isolated vitamin deficiencies, the vitamin in question can be targeted for supplement treatment. The key is to recognize signs of each deficiency by physical examination.

Marasmus

Marasmus causes wasting, emaciation, irritability, and distended abdomen.

Kwashiorkor

Kwashiorkor causes bilateral, pitting limb edema, periorbital edema, desquamation, hair changes, lethargy, and hepatomegaly.

Beriberi (Vitamin B₁ Deficiency)

Deficiency in vitamin B_1 causes neuropathy, limb weakness in dry beriberi, and pronounced swelling in wet beriberi.

Pellagra (Vitamin B₃ Deficiency)

This deficiency causes a classic triad of dermatitis, diarrhea, and dementia. The dermatitis is a photosensitive, sunburn-like rash at sun-exposed sites. There can also be a collar-like ring of scaly skin around the neck known as Casal's necklace. Lesions are sensitive and inflamed, and later they can become scaly and peel off. There are atrophic patches between the fingers, and nails become brittle and atrophic.

Vitamin B₁₂ deficiency

This deficiency can cause hyperpigmentation of the hands and feet, angular stomatitis, as well as blood dyscrasias and neurological abnormalities.

Scurvy (Vitamin C Deficiency)

Scurvy is characterized by swollen, painful joints, dry skin, hyperkeratosis of hair follicles, "corkscrew hairs," bruising, petechial hemorrhage, and dental caries.

Zinc deficiency

Deficiency in zinc can cause scaly lesions on the feet, buttocks, and around the mouth, stunting, developmental delay, recurrent infections, failure to thrive, and persistent diarrhea. [8]

Noninfectious Skin Diseases

Lupus

Lupus erythematosus (LE) occurs mainly in three forms—systemic (acute, visceral), subacute cutaneous (SCLE), and discoid, mainly involving the skin in sun-exposed areas (chronic, cutaneous). Features of lupus include redness of the skin, telangiectasia, hyperpigmentation and hypopigmentation, follicular hyperkeratosis, and atrophy. Several drugs may cause lupus-like symptoms or trigger systemic LE (such as procainamide, isoniazid, hydralazine, and anticonvulsants). In lupus-like drug reactions, symptoms resolve a few weeks after stopping the drug. Patients with LE are often photosensitive, hence the facial butterfly patch rash where the skin is exposed to the sun.

Therapy involves UV barrier protection, oral and topical steroids, immunosuppressants, and hydroxychloroquine. [5]

Stevens-Johnson Syndrome/Toxic Epidermal Necrolysis

Stevens-Johnson syndrome is a systemic disorder with pronounced blistering affecting the oral and genital mucous membranes and the skin. The outcome may be fatal because of dehydration and superimposed sepsis. Serious complications can include corneal ulceration, uveitis, and panophthalmia. Other complications include scarring and adhesions, particularly on the eyelid (synechia). Stevens-Johnson syndrome/toxic epidermal necrolysis is most often caused by a drug reaction, commonly penicillins, sulfa drugs, and HIV medications.

Treatment is with IV fluids to prevent dehydration, Vaseline gauze, removal of offending agents, and pain medications including sedation for severe forms. Daily dressing changes and daily clean sheets are also required. [5]

Opportunistic Infections

Crusted Scabies

Crusted scabies is a diffuse, crusted form of the pruritic scabies mite infection. Scabies is transmitted by direct human-to-human contact and is common in overcrowded conditions. This form of scabies can be found in HIV patients, as well as among elderly and immunocompromised persons. Itching is intense and often worsens at night. Patients shows signs of scratching along with the characteristic scabies burrows and widespread intense, erythematous lichenification, sometimes containing pus. The face is usually spared and the genitals are invariably involved. Other sites commonly involved include the hands, finger webs, nipples, axillae, and inguinal folds.

Treatment requires decontamination of clothing and bedding and several applications of benzyl benzoate or permethrin to the whole skin surface except the head. Oral ivermectin is very effective and be necessary in the crusted variant. Symptomatic relief can be given with topical and systemic antipruritics. [7,9]

Zoster

Zoster is caused by infection with varicella-zoster virus, which causes chickenpox and may subsequently remain dormant in nerve ganglia. With waning immunity or at times of stress or old age, the virus can reactivate, resulting in herpes zoster eruption along the dermatomal distribution of the nerve root. The initial symptom is usually pain with or without burning and/or itching in the nerve-root distribution for up to a week before the lesions erupt. This pain can be severe. Lesions appear as grouped vesicles on an erythematous base. In immunocompromised patients, the eruption can be generalized and highly debilitating.

Treatment involves analgesia, including gabapentin and amitriptyline, povidone-iodine, systemic antiviral agents, oral steroids (only with antivirals for complications), and urgent ophthalmology consult for eye involvement. Pregnant patients and those who have not had chicken pox or been vaccinated for varicella should be kept away from infected individuals or wear protective covering. [5]

Syphilis

Syphilis is a sexually transmitted infection. It has three stages. The primary stage is a painless (usually genital) ulcer. The secondary stage is marked by generalized symptoms of variable severity, such as headache, hoarseness, sore throat, fever, and muscular aching. The rash in the secondary stage consists of raised pink to brown papules and plaques of variable scale. Characteristics of this rash are relatively abrupt onset with involvement of the palms and soles. Hair loss is frequent. The tertiary stage is rare and involves the heart, nervous system, and skin. Skin lesions tend to be annular, with a healing scarred center and slowly advancing outside edge.

Treatment is with penicillin; all exposed partners should be treated. Add probenecid for tertiary-stage syphilis and for patients with AIDS. Use doxycycline for penicillin-allergic patients. [5]

Cutaneous Tuberculosis (TB)

The cutaneous primary complex consists of a tuberculous chancre, lymphangitis, and lymphadenitis. The primary lesion starts as a soft papule, which quickly disintegrates. Lupus vulgaris (cutaneous facial TB) often presents as a destructive, central-facial, verrucous plaque with nasal destruction.

Treatment involves multidrug, prolonged treatment.[5,9]

References

1. Bandino J, Hang A, Norton S. The infectious and noninfectious dermatological consequences of flooding: a field manual for the responding provider. *Am J Clin Dermatol.* 2015;16:399–424.

2. Kc S, Khanal L, Ohja A, Karn D. Diseases in disaster: post-earthquake dermatoses, Nepal 2015. *Kathmandu Univ Med J.* 2016; 55: 279–281.

3. Steigleder G, Maibach H. *Pocket Atlas of Dermatology.* 2nd ed. New York: Thieme Medical Publishers; 1993.

4. Auerbach P, Donner H, Weiss E. *Field Guide to Wilderness Medicine.* 3rd ed. Philadelphia: Mosby Elsevier; 2008.

5. Saxe N, Jessop S, Todd G. *Handbook of Dermatology for Primary Care.* Cape Town: Oxford University Press; 2004.

6. Merriman A, Mwebesa E, Katabira E. *Palliative Medicine: Pain and Symptom Control in the Cancer and/or AIDS Patient in Uganda and other African Countries.* 5th ed. Kampala: Uprise Graphics; 2012.

7. Hay R, Fuller C, Mitjà, Yotsu R, ed. *Recognizing Neglected Tropical Disease Through Changes on the Skin: A Training Guide for Frontline Health Workers.* Geneva: World Health Organization; 2018.

8. Davidson R, Brent A, Seale A, ed. *Oxford Handbook of Tropical Medicine.* 4th ed. Oxford: Oxford University Press; 2014.

9. Basset A, Maleville J, Basset M, Liautaud B. *Infectious and Parasitic Diseases on Black Skin.* London: Science Press Limited; 1988.

Chapter 9

Care of the Dying Patient

Megan Doherty and Joshua Hauser

Introduction

Care of the dying patient generally refers to care in the last days or hours of life. The goals of care during the last hours and days of life are to ensure comfort and dignity. Good palliative care does not hasten death.

In humanitarian settings, where healthcare providers may not have expertise in palliative care, identifying when patients are at this stage of life can be challenging. In addition, during this time, physical symptoms can be difficult to control; the best way to ensure they are well managed is to anticipate the symptoms and develop a management plan.

This chapter will discuss the key physiological changes, communication, and symptom management considerations required to provide care of the dying patient in humanitarian-crisis situations. While providing optimal care for dying patients in these situations may be challenging, a clear understanding of key components of good care can guide clinicians to prioritize their efforts.

Recognizing When Death Is Imminent

When death is approaching, most individuals look quite similar, despite their underlying medical condition. Observations that may help to identify patients who are approaching end of life include the following:

- Very tired and weak, spending the majority of time sleeping or lying down
- Little or no oral intake and difficulty swallowing
- Altered level of consciousness—confused, agitated, restless, or drowsy
- Changes in pulse, blood pressure, and breathing, cool and mottled extremities
- Decreased urine and stool output

Children are often more resilient and may survive what appears to be the imminently dying phase, because they have less age-related degeneration of vital organs. Patients with malnutrition will have a more rapid progression to end of life.

Predicting how long a patient will live is very challenging; changes in the patient's condition should guide prognostication. If changes are:

- Hourly, death is expected in hours to several days.
- Daily, death is expected in days to several weeks.
- Weeks, death is expected in weeks to months.

Ensuring a Good Death

Research indicates that patients and family members feel that a "good death" includes the following[1,2]:

• Communication and clear decision-making from healthcare providers
• Adequate pain and symptom management
• Strengthening relationships with loved ones (resolving conflicts, saying goodbye)
• Preparation for death

Completing these actions may be challenging for clinicians in humanitarian crises. In these settings, when staff might be limited, having a nonmedical member of the healthcare team (such as a patient guide, community health worker, or other staff member) stay with the family can be critical and reduce the family's demands on the healthcare team.

Communication

It is important to provide clear and prompt information about prognosis to the patient and family. When speaking about how much time is left, one should provide a time range, since a precise answer is likely to be wrong and may cause families to lose trust in the clinical team (Box 9.1). Box 9.2 provides suggested language for these conversations.

Box 9.1 Respiratory Pattern Changes

• When talking to families about how long the patient is expected to live, acknowledge uncertainty and always give a time range, for example: "It can be difficult to predict, but I expect that he will live for hours to a few days."

• Be honest about the situation, since this helps families to plan appropriately. For example, ensure that loved ones are present or are aware of the situation.

  • Clear and honest information is valued and preferred.[3]

  • Honesty does not lead to a loss of hope but instead demonstrates your team's honesty and transparency.[4]

  • Avoid saying, "There is nothing more that can be done," as there are always things that can be done, such as treatment of pain and other symptoms.

• Use the checklist in Box 9.2 to guide the conversation when you expect that death is expected soon (adapted from Serious Illness Conversation Guide).[5,6] This sequence follows evidence about the best structure for delivering difficult news and discussing goals of care.

Box 9.2 Key Steps for Conversation to Inform Family that Death is Expected and to Establish Plan of Care

1. Set up the conversation by introducing yourself and asking permission to proceed: "Can I talk to you about what is happening to your loved one?"

2. Assess the family's understanding of the illness: "What is your understanding of where your loved one is at with their illness?"

3. Share the prognosis: "I wish it were different, but I am worried that your loved one is very sick and will not be able to recover from this illness. We do not have any treatments that can cure this problem, and I am worried that your loved one is not going to live for very long."

4. Assess goals and wishes: "What are your goals, given the information I have shared with you?"

5. Establish a plan: "I recommend that we focus on providing care that ensures that your loved one is comfortable, and they can be with those they love."

6. Close the conversation: "We will be here to treat and support your loved one and your family."

Family Meeting Tips

- Sit down and give the patient and family your undivided attention for 5 to 10 minutes, in the most quiet and private location possible and practical for the setting.
- Be honest about how much time you have: "I would really like to spend more time with you, but unfortunately, I only have 10 minutes, so what are the most important questions you have for me at this time?"
- Tell the family when you will be able to return to see them.
- If possible, involve a nurse and psychosocial counselor in the meeting, who can continue to provide support after the meeting.

Symptom Management Considerations in the Last Hours and Day

Guidelines and standardized order sets are recommended to ensure consistent treatment with appropriate doses of medications and to enable bedside clinicians to initiate care. See Box 9.3 for an example.

Ensure that the healthcare team (or family) has the following medications available to be given immediately for severe symptoms (such as pain, dyspnea, and agitation or restlessness) at the end of life.

- Subcutaneous/Intravenous (SC/IV) morphine (or another opioid, if available)
- Rectal (PR) diazepam (or midazolam SC/IV if available)

The goal at this stage is comfort, not to reverse the underlying cause of the symptom. Discontinue vital sign assessments, pulse oximetry, nonessential medications (including IV fluids), and laboratory and radiological tests.

Box 9.3 Suggested Guidelines for Management of Escalating Pain, Dyspnea, and Agitation

Escalating Pain, Dyspnea, and Agitation

No ceiling dose exists for symptom management in the last hours or days of life (end-of-life phase). The correct dose is the dose that relieves the patient's symptoms. Titrate the medications rapidly (over minutes to few hours).

Loading Dose

For patients already on opioids: Administer loading dose of opioid equal to 10% of total dose in past 24 hours

For patients not already on opioids: Administer IV or SC loading dose as follows:

Morphine 5 mg, children <12 years: 0.1 mg/kg

Subsequent Dosing

Doses may be given every 10 minutes PRN for end-of-life symptoms.
Escalate dose as follows (note: 5 mg is given as an example, actual dose may vary):

First dose: 5 mg, if ineffective after 10 minutes, then give

Second dose: 5 mg, if ineffective after 10 minutes, notify prescriber,

Third dose: 7.5 mg (1.5× starting dose), if ineffective, after 10 minutes, then give

Fourth dose: 7.5 mg (1.5× starting dose), if ineffective after 10 minutes, then give

Fifth dose: 10 mg (2× starting dose)

Once good pain relief is achieved, provide the total dose administered during the titration phase SC or IV q4h regularly and as a PRN/SOS dose.

Do not use only PRN doses, as this will allow the symptoms to return and will lead to more distress.

Pain assessment may be by use of pain scale or observations of verbal and non-verbal behavior (crying, grimacing, and moaning either at rest or when moved).

Continuous Infusion Instructions

Recommended hourly rate = total opioid administered in the steps just out-lined, divided by 4.
Recommended 24-hour amount of medication = total opioid administered in the steps just outlined, multiplied by 6.

Adjuvant Therapy for Symptoms that May Accompany Pain or Dyspnea
See Chapter 13 for dosing.

For agitation

Recommended starting dose:

PO//IV/SL/PR lorazepam or PO/SC/IV midazolam: PRN for anxiety or agitation

SC/IV/PO haloperidol: PRN for hallucinations or agitation

For Excess Respiratory Secretions

Oral atropine 1% eye drop solution, SC glycopyrrolate or SC hyoscine butylbromide

Adapted from *Textbook of Interdisciplinary Pediatric Palliative Care.*[8]

If symptoms are not well managed, this suffering may be the family's final memory of their loved one, which can cause further distress and complicated bereavement.

Do not be afraid to rapidly increase the dose of morphine or other medications in order to achieve symptom control. For patients who experience refractory symptoms, palliative sedation can be considered (full details are beyond the scope of this chapter).

The SC route is useful in this phase of illness in order to manage symptoms quickly, without the trouble of needing to maintain IV access. Insert a butterfly needle and secure it in place. This can be kept for up to 7 days (provided the SC site does not have any significant redness or tenderness). Medications that can be given SC (same dose as IV) include the following. See also Chapter 13 for complete details and a compatibility chart.[7]

- **Opioids**: morphine, hydromorphone, fentanyl, methadone, oxycodone, diamorphine
- **Sedative-hypnotics**: midazolam, clonazepam, phenobarbital
- **Antiemetics**: haloperidol, metoclopramide, levomepromazine (methotrimeprazine)
- **Antisecretory agents**: hyoscine butylbromide, hyoscine hydrobromide, glycopyrrolate. octreotide
- **Antihistamines**: cyclizine, promethazine
- **Miscellaneous**: dexamethasone, methylnaltrexone, naloxone

Escalating Pain, Dyspnea, and Agitation

These are three common symptoms that often require intensive treatment near the end of life. The use of rapidly escalating doses of opioids is appropriate to manage pain or dyspnea and, when used by trained providers, will not cause respiratory depression or addiction or hasten death (see Box 9.3).

To facilitate rapid titration of medications, ensure that clinicians are readily available and that medications, including opioids, are available at the bedside for rapid administration. Refer to Chapters 4, 5, and 7 for complete management.

Confusion, Disorientation, and Delirium

Delirium at this stage is generally due to multiple conditions, which are generally irreversible, such as the underlying disease process, metabolic and electrolyte imbalances, liver and renal failure, infection, and hypoxia. Urinary retention is a potentially reversible cause, which can be managed with insertion of a Foley catheter. Refer to Chapter 7 for guidelines in treating delirium.

Counsel the Family

Patients may still be able to hear, so encourage family members to speak to and reassure their loved one.

Weakness and Fatigue

This condition is expected and will increase as the patient gets closer to death. Do not give stimulants (methylphenidate, steroids) to try "to wake the patient up" at this stage of illness. Ensure that the patient is gently turned and repositioned, to avoid pressure ulcers (if death is imminent, this is not relevant).

Counsel the Family

Allow the patient to rest, as weakness and fatigue are a normal part of the dying process. The patient will have a limited amount of energy, so help the patient prioritize how they want to use their energy.

Some patients may experience a brief period of increased energy and mental alertness prior to their death. If this occurs, it should be used for quality interaction with loved ones.

Decreased Oral Intake

Reduced oral intake is a normal part of the dying process; patients who are close to dying do not feel hunger or thirst. Fluids and foods should be provided if desired by the patient. Do not provide parenteral fluids since research shows that this does not improve symptoms, quality of life, or survival for palliative care patients who cannot drink.[9]

Counsel the Family

Forcing a patient to eat or drink may be dangerous because of the risk of aspiration. Providing IV fluids will not prolong life or improve comfort, but it can cause distress from edema and dyspnea. Providing oral care by swabbing the mouth with water and keeping the lips moist with petroleum jelly (Vaseline) or lip balm is recommended.

For families who are struggling with stopping (or not starting IV fluids), a trial of 24 hours of IV/SC fluids may be offered. Discuss with the family and agree on the goals of the therapy. Prior to starting fluids, reassess daily; if the patient is not improving, then discontinue fluids.

Respiration Pattern Changes

Breathing will change as the patient approaches end of life, with breathing becoming slow and shallow or rapid and shallow. Periods of apnea or increased work of breathing are common but do not necessarily indicate dyspnea, and need not be treated unless it is distressing to the patient.

Counsel the Family

Advise the family that breathing changes may occur, but generally do not cause distress in the patient.

Respiratory Secretions

Patients often have impaired ability to swallow at the end of life and cannot clear secretions. These secretions can accumulate and lead to gurgling or rattling sounds. This most often occurs when the patient is only minimally conscious or unconscious and does not cause the patient any distress.

Position the patient on their side with the upper body elevated to allow secretions to passively drain out of the mouth. Reduce or stop artificial (IV) fluids or nutrition (IV or NG), since this will worsen this symptom.

Suctioning is not usually helpful and may be distressing to the patient. Consider suctioning only if thick mucus or blood is present in the mouth and can easily be removed with a soft catheter.

Medications

- Atropine 1% (eye drop solution), glycopyrrolate, hyoscine butylbromide, or hyoscine hydrobromide

The following medications will not work for secretions deep in the lungs (i.e., pulmonary edema or pneumonia) and are not always effective for upper airway secretions. See Chapter 13 for dosing.

Counsel the Family

Convey to the family that the patient is unaware of this symptom and it is not causing them discomfort.

Incontinence and Urinary Retention

Incontinence of urine, stool, or both is common. Keep the patient clean and dry. A Foley catheter may be helpful but is not always needed, since urine output is minimal and absorbent pads or cloth and plastic can be used.

Urinary retention may occur and should be suspected in a restless patient with a distended bladder. In this case, a Foley catheter should be inserted.

Urinary retention can be a side effect of opioid medication, which is more commonly seen in infants and young children. A Foley catheter or intermittent catheterization may be needed.

Seizures and Convulsions

Seizures can be caused by cancers (primary or metastatic), drug toxicity (e.g., pethidine/meperidine), metabolic or electrolyte abnormalities (hypoglycemia, hyponatremia, hypercalcemia), hypoxia, severe liver failure, infections of the central nervous system (CNS), or epilepsy. Treatment is comfort focused, and a full investigative workup is not necessary.

For children with a history of epilepsy, if the child can no longer swallow medications, SC midazolam or another benzodiazepine should be started.

Management
See Chapter 13 for dosing. Corticosteroids can be considered for seizures secondary to brain metastasis, to reduce peritumoral edema.

Acute Treatment (Status Epilepticus)
- **Diazepam, lorazepam,** or **midazolam,** repeat after 5 or 10 minutes if needed.
- If these are ineffective, consider doubling the dose of midazolam or diazepam or give **phenobarbital**.
- This should be followed with regular phenobarbital, to prevent further seizures.

Prophylactic Management
- This should only be considered for patients with brain metastasis who have already had a seizure or malignant melanoma with brain metastases and in children with epilepsy.
- Phenytoin, carbamazepine, or valproate can be considered.

Pediatric Treatment Considerations
Parents should be trained in the use of sublingual (SL) lorazepam or rectal (PR) diazepam as abortive medications if a child is likely to have a prolonged seizure at home. Box 9.4 provides guidance on PR administration as an alternative route.

Box 9.4 Rectal Administration of Medications for Children

Administer medication rectally in children using a syringe attached to a small feeding tube cut to 5 cm in length. Insert the feeding tube 4 to 5 cm beyond the anal margin for an older child and less for an infant.

Home-Based Palliative Care

Families should be asked about their preferred location for death. Providing home-based palliative care in a humanitarian crisis is possible and, indeed, preferable, as it may relieve the burden on healthcare facilities. Several home-based palliative care services have been developed in refugee camps and other humanitarian crisis situations.[10,11]

For patients who wish to go home, it is very important to provide a 24-hour contact number for a clinician, since families frequently need advice about symptom management. Without telephone support, patients frequently return to the hospital when pain or other symptoms are not well controlled or they die at home with significant suffering.

Providing home visits from trained community health workers enables families to stay at home. Counseling and training for family caregivers prior to discharge is important. Box 9.5 shows a checklist for counseling caregivers preparing for death at home.[12]

Home palliative care team members should include the following:

- Community health workers (CHW) with training in basic home-based palliative care
- Physicians and nurses with training in palliative care who supervise and provide guidance to the CHWs and visit patients who are having significant uncontrolled symptoms

---

Box 9.5 Counseling Checklist for Family Caregivers

Physical Care

- Moisten mouth with ice chips or a damp cloth soaked in water or fruit juice.
- Keep lips moist with balm or petroleum jelly (Vaseline).
- Keep the person clean and dry; use cloths or pads for urinary incontinence.
- Give the medications to control symptoms, at the correct times.
- Do not wait until the symptoms are severe, as this will lead to symptoms that are more difficult to control.
- Do not force the person to eat or drink. If they do not want to eat, this is okay.
- Assist the person to change position or turn every 2 hours to prevent pressure ulcers.
- Contact the home palliative care team (or whoever is providing 24-hour telephone support) if pain or other symptoms are not controlled.

Emotional and Spiritual Care

- Tell the person that they are loved and will be remembered.
- Ensure that the person has opportunities to discuss any feelings of guilt, worry, or regret.
- Connect with spiritual or religious leaders if the person wishes this.
- Sit with the person, hold their hand, and talk to them.

An emergency symptom management kit, kept at the patient's home, can be used by CHW or trained family members to provide relief for acute distress in a patient at the end of life. The kit should contain the following medications:

• Morphine (or other opioid)—for pain and dyspnea
• Haloperidol—for nausea and delirium
• Hyoscine butylbromide (or other agent for oral secretions/congestion)—for secretions
• Midazolam, diazepam (or other benzodiazepine)— for seizures, catastrophic bleeding, and acute respiratory distress

Special Situations

Unsuccessful Resuscitation

During resuscitation, allowing the family to be present is preferred, as this can lead to less anxiety, depression, and second-guessing about the care provided and the competence of staff.[13,14]

A member of the healthcare team should be assigned to stay with the family to update them about what is happening, answer their questions, and provide emotional support.

Discontinuing Fluids and Nutrition

In patients who have hours or days to live, it is considered standard of care to discontinue medically administered fluids and nutrition (see section Decreased Oral Intake).

Medically provided fluids and nutrition can ethically be withheld or withdrawn if they are no longer in the best interest of the patient—for example, if they only prolong and add morbidity to the process of dying.[15] Fluids and nutrition may be withdrawn from a child who permanently lacks awareness and the ability to interact with the environment, such as a child in a persistent vegetative state or children with anencephaly.

It is important to counsel patients and families that this does not mean clinicians are "giving up" on a patient or abandoning the patient but rather focusing intensely on comfort and support.

Discontinuing Ventilatory Support

It may be ethically appropriate to discontinue intensive respiratory support (e.g., noninvasive or invasive ventilation) in certain circumstances. These supports are often started when a patient's prognosis or illness trajectory is unclear or when the patient is believed to have a reversible condition.

It may become clear that the underlying cause of ventilator dependence is irreversible. In these situations, continued ventilatory support will not provide meaningful quality of life and may prolong suffering. This act of discontinuing ventilator support (or other life-sustaining treatments) is not the same as euthanasia or medical assistance in dying.

It is essential to involve the family in the decision to discontinue ventilatory support. Involving religious or cultural leaders may also be necessary.

After discontinuation of ventilation, most patients live only minutes or hours; however, there are some patients who may live for a few days or longer. Clinicians must prepare the family for the possibility that the individual may breathe on their own, especially in pediatrics, where this is more common.[16]

Management: Before Withdrawing Ventilator

- Ensure that family are present, if desired.
- Turn off all monitors and alarms.
- Discontinue all other life-sustaining treatments (e.g., artificial nutrition and hydration, antibiotics, dialysis).
- Remove all unnecessary medical paraphernalia (NG tubes, IV lines, etc.).
- Allow any neuromuscular blocking agents to wear off.
- Ensure that a rapid-acting opioid (e.g., morphine), benzodiazepine (e.g., midazolam or lorazepam), and an agent to manage secretions (e.g., glycopyrrolate) are available and drawn up at the patient's bedside.
- Give a dose of opioids and benzodiazepine prior to withdrawing the ventilator, to ensure the patient does not feel any discomfort or dyspnea.[17]

Process of Withdrawal

- Ensure that the patient appears comfortable.
- Withdrawal by immediate extubation is recommended.[18]

After Ventilator Withdrawal

- If the patient appears distressed, symptoms should be immediately and aggressively controlled, by giving morphine and midazolam, every 10 minutes, until distress is relieved.
- A clinician should be easily available to answer questions and manage symptoms.

Memory Making

While this is especially relevant parents when a child dies, it can also be meaningful for families of an adult who dies. Having tangible objects to remember their loved one supports the family in their grief. This is especially important with a pregnancy or infant loss, as parents have few tangible memories of their child's short life.

In many cultures, parents are encouraged to try to quickly forget that a child has died, but this is not recommended, as it leads to more complicated grief for parents.

Having tangible objects to remember their loved one supports the family in their grief. This is especially important with a pregnancy or infant loss, as parents have few tangible memories of their child's short life.

Common memory-making activities that can be easily offered to families include the following:

- Photographs or videos.
- Prints or molds of hands and feet, locks of hair

- Linking objects, which provide a physical reminder of the connection between the child and loved one (e.g., a pair of special necklaces or bracelets, one of which is placed with the child and the other with the parent).
- Personal items: clothing, baby blanket, small toys, hospital bracelet, birth certificate, bassinet card.
- Memory boxes: items can be stored and looked at when desired.

Some parents may not want to keep any memory items, which should be respected. All parents should be offered memory making, since in all cultures, there are some parents who will desire this.[19]

After-Death Care

It is important to express empathy with a simple statement, such as "I am sorry for your loss." Confirm the death by physical examination (absence of heart sounds, palpable pulse, or respirations for 60 seconds). Document the date and time of death in the medical record and the cause of death.

Allow the family as much time as they desire to say goodbye and to perform any religious or cultural rituals, as permitted within the limitations of the setting.

During an epidemic (e.g., Ebola), it may not be possible to release the body to the family, so assistance from a psychologist or spiritual support person is important to support the family's bereavement.

Supporting Staff Who Provide End-of-Life Care

Witnessing frequent suffering and death can cause staff burnout, compassion fatigue, and moral distress. Chapter 17 provides more details about how to address this.

Regular support meetings create a safe space for staff to reflect and express their emotions on providing end-of-life care. Staff can reflect on the care that was delivered—what went well, what could be improved. Senior staff members should attend to demonstrate the importance of seeking support.

Commemorating the patient is also important for healthcare providers. This can be done by having memorial services, attending funeral services, or having follow-up contact with families. Letters, phone calls, or text messages from staff are deeply valued by families who often treasure the memories of this small act of kindness by staff.[20]

References

1. Pierson CM, Curtis JR, Patrick DL. A good death: A qualitative study of patients with advanced AIDS. *AIDS Care*. 2002;14(5):587–598. doi:10.1080/0954012021000005416

2. Steinhauser KE, Clipp EC, McNeilly M, Christakis NA, McIntyre LM, Tulsky JA. In search of a good death: observations of patients, families, and providers. *Ann Intern Med*. 2000;132(10):825. doi:10.7326/0003-4819-132-10-200005160-00011

3. Mack JW, Smith TJ. Reasons why physicians do not have discussions about poor prognosis, why it matters, and what can be improved. *J Clin Oncol.* 2012;30(22):2715–2717.

4. Meyer EC, Ritholz MD, Burns JP, Truog RD. Improving the quality of end-of-life care in the pediatric intensive care unit: parents' priorities and recommendations. *Pediatrics.* 2006;117(3):649–657. doi:10.1542/peds.2005-0144

5. Bernacki RE, Block SD. Communication about serious illness care goals: a review and synthesis of best practices. *JAMA Intern Med.* 2014;174(12):1994–2003. doi:10.1001/jamainternmed.2014.5271

6. Bernacki R, Hutchings M, Vick J, et al. Development of the Serious Illness Care Program: a randomised controlled trial of a palliative care communication intervention. *BMJ Open.* 2015;5(10):e009032. doi:10.1136/bmjopen-2015-009032

7. Jassal SS. *Basic Symptom Control in Paediatric Palliative Care: The Rainbows Children's Hospice Guidelines.* 9th ed. Bristol, UK: Together for Short Lives; 2013. http:// www.icpcn.org/wp-content/uploads/2013/09/Rainbows-Basic-Symptom-Control-In-Paediatric-Palliative-Care-Ninth-Edition-PDF.pdf. Accessed June 29, 2019.

8. Wolfe J, Hinds P, Sourkes B. *Textbook of Interdisciplinary Pediatric Palliative Care.* St. Louis: Elsevier; 2011.

9. Bruera E, Hui D, Dalal S, et al. Parenteral hydration in patients with advanced cancer: a multicenter, double-blind, placebo-controlled randomized trial. *J Clin Oncol.* 2013;31(1):111–118. doi:10.1200/JCO.2012.44.6518

10. Doherty M, Khan, F. Neglected Suffering: The Unmet Need for Palliative Care in Cox's Bazar. https://reliefweb.int/report/bangladesh/neglected-suffering-unmet-need-palliative-care-cox-s-bazar. Accessed April 11, 2018.

11. Pinheiro I, Jaff D. The role of palliative care in addressing the health needs of Syrian refugees in Jordan. *Med Confl Surviv.* 2018;34(1):19–38. doi:10.1080/13623699.2018.1437966

12. World Health Organization (WHO). *Palliative Care: Symptom Management and End-of-Life Care—Interim Guidelines for First-Level Facility Health Workers.* Geneva: World Health Organization; 2004. https://www.who.int/hiv/pub/imai/primary_palliative/en/. Accessed February 13, 2019.

13. Nibert L, Ondrejka D. Family presence during pediatric resuscitation: an integrative review for evidence-based practice. *J Pediatr Nurs.* 2005;20(2):145–147. doi:10.1016/j.pedn.2004.05.017

14. Jabre P, Belpomme V, Azoulay E, et al. Family presence during cardiopulmonary resuscitation. *N Engl J Med.* 2013;368(11):1008–1018. doi:10.1056/NEJMoa1203366

15. Tsai E; Canadian Paediatric Society, Bioethics Committee. Withholding and withdrawing artificial nutrition and hydration. *Paediatr Child Health.* 2011;16(4):241–242. https://www.cps.ca/en/documents/position/withholding-withdrawing-artificial-nutrition-hydration. Accessed July 12, 2018.

16. von Gunten C, Weissman DE. Information for patients and families about ventilator withdrawal #35. *J Palliat Med.* 2003;6(5):775–776. doi:10.1089/109662103322515310

17. von Gunten C, Weissman DE. Symptom control for ventilator withdrawal in the dying patient #34. *J Palliat Med.* 2003;6(5):774–775. doi:10.1089/109662103322515301

18. von Gunten C, Weissman DE. Ventilator withdrawal protocol (part I) #33. *J Palliat Med.* 2003;6(5):773–774. doi:10.1089/109662103322515293

19. Cortezzo DE, Sanders MR, Brownell EA, Moss K. End-of-life care in the neonatal intensive care unit: experiences of staff and parents. *Am J Perinatol*. 2015;32(8):713–724. doi:10.1055/s-0034-1395475

20. Macdonald ME. Parental perspectives on hospital staff members' acts of kindness and commemoration after a child's death. *Pediatrics*. 2005;116(4):884–890. doi:10.1542/peds.2004-1980

Chapter 10

Noncommunicable Diseases in Crisis Regions

Sujatha Sankaran, Sriram Shamasunder, Marcia Glass, and Mhoira E.F. Leng

Cardiomyopathies

General Principles of Symptom Management

Cardiomyopathies are diseases that impair cardiac function and can be caused by ischemic as well as nonischemic injuries to the heart. There are many etiologies that lead to impairment in the pumping function of the heart, and most of those listed here lead to a dilatation of the heart. But, regardless of etiology, symptomatic management is often the same.[1] Etiologies of cardiomyopathy include coronary artery disease leading to ischemic cardiomyopathy, peripartum cardiomyopathy, hypertrophic cardiomyopathy, amyloid cardiomyopathy, alcohol-induced cardiomyopathy, HIV-associated cardiomyopathy, and trypanosomiasis.[2] The primary focus of symptomatic treatment is on reducing symptoms of volume overload and optimizing cardiac output to alleviate dyspnea and fatigue.

Nonpharmacological Symptom Management

Volume overload in patients with cardiomyopathy can cause dyspnea, orthopnea, and generalized fatigue. A limit of 2 g sodium daily is appropriate, but this can be difficult to quantify for many patients. The patient should also be educated about other sources of salt, such as prepackaged food, sauces, and canned foods. Exertion is often limited in these patients because of fatigue and dyspnea.[3]

Pharmacological Symptom Management

Volume overload in patients with cardiomyopathies can initially be treated with a loop diuretic such as furosemide, bumetanide, or torsemide, in combination with dietary salt restriction.[4] A pharmacological regimen for cardiomyopathy includes a beta blocker and aspirin for all patients without contraindications, in addition to management of volume overload in appropriate patients.[5] Other therapies that may be appropriate in some patients are the combination of hydralazine and a nitrate and mineralocorticoid receptor antagonists such as spironolactone or eplerenone.[6]

Dementia

General Principles of Symptom Management

Mental health is an often neglected area of noncommunicable diseases (see Chapters 7 and 16 in this book for coverage of adjustment disorder, anxiety, trauma, and delirium), and chronic and acute psychotic illness may be missed in a humanitarian setting. Patients with these symptoms may be subjected to stigma and cultural misinterpretation. People living with learning difficulties may also be vulnerable. It is thus important to work closely with mental health workers for patients' wider needs.

Dementia is a general term that encompasses a number of pathological processes and refers to the loss of cognitive functioning and behavior that results in an inability to carry out one's activities of daily living. Affected patients have trouble with thinking, memory, language, reasoning, and problem-solving, in addition to emotional dysregulation that can cause personality changes.[7] As the severity of dementia increases, people become unable to carry out basic activities of daily living. Dementia has become increasingly common in resource-limited settings; life expectancy in these regions has increased, and dementia accompanies primarily diseases of aging.[8] Dementia treatment is mainly symptomatic and involves manipulation of the physical environment to support patient safety and functioning.

Nonpharmacological Symptom Management

In patients with dementia, it is important to consider the sociocultural situation and to determine who the surrogate decision-makers are. In advanced dementia, the patient's next of kin or closest friends will have to serve as surrogate decision-makers. It is important to make them aware of this and ensure that ethical and legal implications are addressed for decision-making, management of assets, and other responsibilities. Open discussion with decision-makers will be important as the patient's illness progresses. The patient and caregivers should be aware that as the illness progresses, the patient will not be able to report side effects to therapy and fully participate in treatment decisions, so these issues should be discussed at the outset of diagnosis. The patient and caregiver should discuss whether the patient is interested in focusing on comfort only or also seeks interventions that may be uncomfortable but could prolong life. This discussion should factor in the patient's culture and personal values, what is available, and the place of preferred care.[9]

Impaired eating is a common issue in patients with dementia. Patients with dementia often have a decreased sense of smell, which leads to decreased appetite. Sometimes altering the texture or flavor of the meal can help overcome this issue. Offering small meals high in caloric intake is one approach to maintain nutrition in patients with dementia. Patients with advanced dementia often cannot feed themselves and require hand-feeding. In resource-limited regions, artificial feeding may not be available, but if it is available, it is important to discuss with patients that artificial feeding may impair quality of life and that there is no evidence that it can actually prolong length of life.[10]

Impaired sleep is another issue that patients with dementia can encounter. Nonpharmacological approaches to insomnia are recommended. These include sleep hygiene techniques, such as avoiding caffeine later in the day, using the bed only for sleep, sleeping in a quiet and dark area, and avoiding alcohol intake.[11]

Cirrhosis

General Principles of Symptom Management

Cirrhosis refers to irreversible end-stage fibrosis of the liver and is the result of a number of pathological processes, including chronic hepatitis B infection, chronic hepatitis C infection, alcohol use, and nonalcoholic steatohepatitis.[12] Cirrhosis can cause a number of debilitating symptoms and complications that themselves produce much morbidity. The general goals of symptomatic treatment of cirrhosis are to address the symptom burden while preventing and treating complications of cirrhosis.[13] Some areas are rolling out vaccinations programs for hepatitis B and antiviral agents, so it is important to be aware of the local resources.

Symptom Management

The most common debilitating symptom of cirrhosis is ascites. Patients with discomfort associated with the ascites should be given a diuretic regimen with furosemide and spironolactone. It is also important for patients with cirrhosis to limit their daily sodium intake to 2000 mg daily.[14] Caution should be exercised with this regimen, as overdiuresis can cause renal insufficiency and place the patient at risk for hepatorenal syndrome. It may also make the patient hypotensive and liable to falls. If the patient is not able to achieve sufficient comfort through diuresis, paracentesis may be indicated to help alleviate ascites symptoms. Paracentesis involves inserting a needle into the peritoneum to drain ascitic liquid. The procedure is relatively safe, even in patients with coagulopathies. As much as 5 to 8 L fluid may be removed during paracentesis, leading to decreased intra-abdominal pressure. Patients with greater than 5 L of fluid removed should be given 6 to 8 g albumin per liter of fluid removed, but, more commonly, smaller amounts are removed, to avoid the need for very expensive albumin.[15]

Management of Complications of Cirrhosis

Muscle cramping is a common symptom of cirrhosis. Other causes of muscle cramps should be excluded and electrolytes should be repleted. If the cramping is severe, quinine sulfate may be administered for symptomatic relief. If quinine is not available, branched-chain amino acids, taurine, or vitamin E can be used.[16]

Another complication of cirrhosis is umbilical hernia. If the hernia is not incarcerated or ruptured, watchful waiting is a reasonable approach, given the high complication rate of surgical repair. Abdominal binders can help alleviate symptoms of the hernia. Chronic hyponatremia is also common and may be caused by treatment with diuretics. Fluid restriction is recommended in patients with sodium levels less than 120 mmol/L.

Esophageal varices caused by pressure building up through the portal venous system are a serious complication, leading to dangerous upper gastrointestinal bleeding. Beta blockers are indicated in patients with cirrhosis for primary and secondary prophylaxis of variceal hemorrhage but should be used with caution in patients with refractory ascites or current spontaneous bacterial peritonitis. If there is access to endoscopy, this should be sought early as part of disease management.

Spontaneous bacterial peritonitis is an infection in the ascitic fluid that can cause abdominal pain and fevers. Management involves treatment with an antibiotic. Hepatic encephalopathy is another complication of cirrhosis that can be life-threatening. Management includes use of lactulose and rifaximin.[17]

Chronic Kidney Disease (CKD)

General Principles of Symptom Management

There is an estimated overall prevalence of 8–16% of CKD around the world.[18] This corresponds to nearly 500 million affected individuals, of whom 78% (387.5 million) reside in low-income to middle-income countries (LMICs). The rate of CKD progression is variable and dependent on the underlying etiology. There are many etiologies which cause CKD, with the largest prevalence being diabetes and high blood pressure. Other etiologies include HIV and other infectious diseases. As CKD is caused by other large groups of medical comorbidities and exposures, there is a three-pronged approach that may be helpful in LMIC:

(1) Treat noncommunicable diseases, including hypertension and diabetes mellitus.

(2) Reduce exposure to environmental toxins, including, pesticides and environmental heavy metals, and provide safe drinking water.

(3) Address and treat infectious diseases including malaria, HIV, hepatitis B and C.[19]

Nonpharmacological Management

CKD stages 1–3 are largely asymptomatic. In CKD stages 4 and 5, patients generally begin to develop symptoms. Fluid management for volume overload can be addressed with decreased salt intake. Malnutrition in CKD is a challenge, and providing enough protein with a low potassium focus is beneficial. Characterizing and avoiding foods that have high potassium are also important. Patients should take less calcium and less phosphate as their kidney failure progresses. Inorganic phosphate has much higher bioavailability than does organic phosphate, therefore, sources rich in inorganic phosphate, such as highly processed foods, should be avoided as much as possible. Protein should be restricted slightly, to a level of 0.8 g/kg/day, in non-nephrotic patients.[20]

Pharmacological Management

Glomerular diseases should be suspected early when patients present with typical clinical and urinary features, such as body swelling, rash, proteinuria, and hematuria.

Blood pressure control to a goal of 140/80 is important. Angiotensin-converting enzyme (ACE) inhibitors are recommended, though some increase in creatinine or hyperkalemia can occur. Diuretics should be used to manage volume status.[21] Correction of metabolic acidosis with bicarbonate is useful, as is using a statin to reduce vascular events.[22] Caution is warranted regarding prescribing medications, as many require a dose reduction in the setting of renal impairment.

Access to renal replacement therapies including dialysis is very limited in most low-resource settings. The decision to start such therapy should be done with care in CKD and working with experts in renal disease.

Malignancies

In crisis areas, there is often no available medical treatment other than trauma management and infection control. For patients with malignancies, this usually means no access to chemotherapy, immunotherapy, radiation, disease-modifying surgeries, or even symptom management. If patients with cancer are unable to travel to other settings for treatment, the best approach is to focus on good palliative care with a holistic approach, including symptom support and excellent communication. The following cancer-related symptoms are explored in these chapters:

Chapter 4: pain

Chapter 5: dyspnea

Chapter 6: nausea and constipation

Chapter 7: delirium and anxiety

Chapter 8: skin care (including pruritus and care of fungating tumors)

Chapter 9: care of the dying patient

Chapter 11: palliative care emergencies (including bleeding, effusions, seizures, SVC syndrome, and spinal cord compression)

Chapter 14: communicating difficult news

References

1. Hunt SA, Abraham WT, Chin MH, et al. 2009 focused update incorporated into the ACC/AHA 2005 guidelines for the diagnosis and management of heart failure in adults: a report of the American College of Cardiology Foundation/American Heart Association Task Force on Practice Guidelines developed in collaboration with the International Society for Heart and Lung Transplantation. *J Am Coll Cardiol.* 2009;53(15):e1–e90.

2. Felker GM, Thompson RE, Hare JM, et al. Underlying causes and long-term survival in patients with initially unexplained cardiomyopathy. *N Engl J Med.* 2000;342(15):1077–1084.

3. Dickson VV, Riegel B. Are we teaching what patients need to know? Building skills in heart failure self-care. *Heart Lung.* 2009;38(3):253–261.

4. Wexler R, Elton T, Pleister A, Feldman D. Cardiomyopathy: an overview. *Am Fam Physician.* 2009;79(9):778.

5. McMurray JJ, Adamopoulos S, Anker SD, et al. ESC guidelines for the diagnosis and treatment of acute and chronic heart failure 2012: the Task Force for the Diagnosis and Treatment of Acute and Chronic Heart Failure 2012 of the European Society of Cardiology. Developed in collaboration with the Heart Failure Association (HFA) of the ESC. *Eur J Heart Failure.* 2012;14(8):803–869.

6. Mant J, Al-Mohammad A, Swain S, Laramée P. Management of chronic heart failure in adults: synopsis of the National Institute for Health and Clinical Excellence guideline. *Ann Intern Med.* 2011;155(4):252–259.

7. Prince M, Bryce R, Albanese E, Wimo A, Ribeiro W, Ferri CP. The global prevalence of dementia: a systematic review and meta-analysis. *Alzheimer Dement.* 2013;9(1):63–75.

8. Kalaria RN, Maestre GE, Arizaga R, et al. Alzheimer's disease and vascular dementia in developing countries: prevalence, management, and risk factors. *Lancet Neurol.* 2008;7(9):812–826.

9. Volicer L. Goals of care in advanced dementia: quality of life, dignity and comfort. *J Nutr Health Aging.* 2007;11(6):481.

10. Volkert D, Chourdakis M, Faxen-Irving G, et al. ESPEN guidelines on nutrition in dementia. *Clin Nutr.* 2015;34(6):1052–1073.

11. Bombois S, Derambure P, Pasquier F, Monaca C. Sleep disorders in aging and dementia. *J Nutr Health Aging.* 2010;14(3):212–217.

12. Perz JF, Armstrong GL, Farrington LA, Hutin YJ, Bell BP. The contributions of hepatitis B virus and hepatitis C virus infections to cirrhosis and primary liver cancer worldwide. *J Hepatol.* 2006;45(4):529–538.

13. Ginès P, Cárdenas A, Arroyo V, Rodés J. Management of cirrhosis and ascites. *N Engl J Med.* 2004;350(16):1646–1654.

14. Gauthier A, Levy VG, Quinton A, et al. Salt or no salt in the treatment of cirrhotic ascites: a randomised study. *Gut.* 1986;27(6):705–709.

15. Ginès P, Titó L, Arroyo V, et al. Randomized comparative study of therapeutic paracentesis with and without intravenous albumin in cirrhosis. *Gastroenterology.* 1988;94(6):1493–1502.

16. Vidot H, Carey S, Allman-Farinelli M, Shackel N. Systematic review: the treatment of muscle cramps in patients with cirrhosis. *Aliment Pharmacol Ther.* 2014;40(3):221–232.

17. Schuppan D, Afdhal NH. Liver cirrhosis. *Lancet.* 2008;371(9615):838–851.

18. Nugent RA, Fathima SF, Feigl AB, Chyung D. The burden of chronic kidney disease on developing nations: a 21st century challenge in global health. *Nephron Clin Pract.* 2011;118:c269–c277. doi: 10.1159/000321382

19. Stanifer WJ, et al. Chronic kidney disease in low- and middle-income countries *Nephrol Dial Transplant.* 2016;31(6):868–874.

20. Garg AX, Blake PG, Clark WF, Clase CM, Haynes RB, Moist LM. Association between renal insufficiency and malnutrition in older adults: results from the NHANES III. *Kidney Int.* 2001;60(5):1867–1874.

21. Klahr S, Levey AS, Beck GJ, et al. The effects of dietary protein restriction and blood-pressure control on the progression of chronic renal disease. *N Engl J Med.* 1994;330:877–884.

22. Vassalotti JA, Centor R, Turner BJ, et al. Practical approach to detection and management of chronic kidney disease for the primary care clinician. *Am J Med.* 2016;129(2):153–162.

Chapter 11

Palliative Care Emergencies in Humanitarian Crises

David M. Williscroft

Introduction

Delivering palliative care in the midst of a humanitarian crisis poses numerous challenges, among them being the provision of acute care during a palliative emergency. These emergencies may differ from those encountered in typical hospital or hospice environments outside of resource challenged zones. Potential emergencies include bleeding, pneumothorax, pleural and pericardial effusions, seizures, superior vena cava (SVC) syndrome and malignant spinal cord compression. The goal of this chapter is to provide some guidance in the approach to and management of these urgencies in the context of limited access to diagnostic and therapeutic tools.

Bleeding

Bleeding is commonly encountered in humanitarian crises, but in the context of treating patients on a palliative trajectory (end-stage cancer, liver disease), the management of these clinical situations may be challenging. Bleeding may occur in the range of 10–15% of patients with cancer alone.[1] The presence of a brisk bleeding episode is usually quite distressing to the patient, family, and caregivers. Understanding the patients' wishes for their care and their prognosis will assist the practitioners in their approach. Utilizing techniques that are accessible, inexpensive, and easy to use will be paramount in the care of active bleeding.[2]

Causes of bleeding may include tumor invasion, thrombocytopenia, carotid blowout syndrome, gastrointestinal sources (such as esophageal varices, ulcers, diverticulosis), nutritional deficiencies (vitamin K, folate, vitamin B_{12}), medications (anticoagulants, antiplatelet agents), and treatment side effects (from radio- and chemotherapy, graft versus host disease).

Depending on the availability of resources and time constraints, the workup may be quite limited. Identifying reversible causes of bleeding such as medications (Coumadin) or bloodline pathologies (disseminated intravascular coagulation, thrombocytopenia, leukemia) may be possible depending on the situation.

Acute presentation of a bleeding emergency may present as epistaxis, decrease in level of consciousness due to intracranial hemorrhage, hemoptysis, hematemesis, melena, hematochezia, vaginal bleeding, hematuria, cutaneous bleeding from wounds or tumors, or internally (thoracic, peritoneal, retroperitoneal).[3]

Management of the bleeding emergency will depend on several factors, including the patient's goals of care and the trajectory of their disease process. Clear communication to the patient and family is a priority in these situations, as the patient may decline within minutes. Having a stated plan will enable the opportunity for the patient to be optimally supported. This may be as basic as providing a private area with suction, dark towels (to offset the visual stress of the blood), and medications for pain and sedation (SC/IV benzodiazepine, opiate, or both), in addition to psychosocial support. For detailed information on medication and dosing for pain associated with bleeding, please refer to Chapters 4, 9, and 13 of this book.

Other potential bleeding scenarios and their management are as follows:

Bleeding wounds: Consider topical epinephrine, tranexamic or aminocaproic acid (powder, IV), direct pressure dressings, cautery (silver nitrate, thermal), and over-sewing small blood vessels.

Brisk hemoptysis: Position patient in lateral decubitus with the affected side (e.g., bronchial tumor) down. Consider radiotherapy, if appropriate, once the patient is stable.

Hematemesis/vaginal bleeding/melena: Attempt to slow rate of blood loss with a trial of tranexamic acid 500–1000 mg (IV/SC/topical with packing).

Medication reversal: If applicable, assess for reversal of agents causing bleeding (e.g., vitamin K, fresh frozen plasma for Coumadin).

Systemic options:

- Octreotide (variceal bleeding)
- Vasopressin infusion
- Antifibrinolytics (tranexamic and aminocaproic acid)
- Platelet transfusion (thrombocytopenia)

Pneumothorax/Pleural and Pericardial Effusions

Dyspnea is a common presenting symptom in patients with palliative needs. Sources of dyspnea may present in a patient in crisis that requires rapid assessment and treatment. The workup of these patients will hinge on the availability of resources (e.g., diagnostic imaging) and other factors, such as rate of deterioration. The approach to caring for the patient in distress will, of course, be dictated by the patient's wishes for care and the discrete clinical scenario. For details regarding medications and dosing, please refer to Chapters 5 and 13.

Pneumothorax/Pleural Effusion

Patients with cancer and non-cancer diagnoses (e.g., COPD or heart failure) may be in distress due to either or both of these lung pathologies. Having a high clinical suspicion for these conditions will help direct the practitioner to address the problem quickly. The diagnosis can be made clinically (history and physical exam) and with the assistance of diagnostic tools, if available. Point-of-care ultrasound

(POCUS)[4] is increasingly being used as an extension of the physical exam in the assessment of patients with dyspnea. The portability, ease of use, and lower cost have made POCUS a reasonable option for many practitioners in resource-poor environments. Ultrasound can help direct the diagnosis and facilitate safe procedures (thoracentesis and tube thoracostomy placement).[5] Traditional modalities, including X-ray and computed tomography (CT) are often not accessible in humanitarian disasters, owing to cost, electricity limitations, and personnel. If applicable, safe placement of tube thoracostomy, thoracentesis, or both may relieve dyspnea and hypoxia in patients in distress.

Pericardial Effusions

Pericardial effusions (PCE) can complicate many disease processes such as cancer (malignant effusion with breast, thyroid cancers), infections (viral, bacterial, parasitic, tuberculosis), metabolic and endocrine disorders (uremia, hypothyroidism), post–myocardial infarction (MI) (Dressler's), and others (trauma, connective tissue disease). Clinical assessment can include Beck's triad (muffled heart sounds, elevated jugular venous pressure [JVP], hypotension) and pulsus paradoxus. POCUS may assist in the diagnosis (transthoracic or subxiphoid views) and treatment (pericardiocentesis +/- pericardial window). Utilization of simple tools such as long spinal needles may be an option where expensive pericardiocentesis kits are not available.

Seizures

In the context of patients with a palliative diagnosis, seizures are not uncommon. They may be due to intracranial metastases or hemorrhage, meningoencephalitis, metabolic abnormalities, or drug overdose, withdrawal, or interactions. Seizures may be generalized or focal, or both. Sustained seizure activity meets the definition of status epilepticus after 5 minutes of generalized or 30 minutes of focal convulsions. The diagnosis can be confirmed with electroencephalogram (EEG) studies, but this is often not a practical approach in a humanitarian-crisis scenario.

The treatment options are largely anchored on cessation via the utilization of benzodiazepines, which are inexpensive and accessible.[6] For further details on medications and dosing, please refer to Chapter 13. Common options include the following:

Midazolam can be administered via multiple routes (IV/SC/buccal/intranasal). Its advantage is rapid onset and duration of action (2.5 hours half-life [t1/2]).

Lorazepam has a longer duration of action than midazolam (t1/2 10–15 hours) with an onset of approximately 3 minutes.

Diazepam may have a more rapid onset than lorazepam because of its ability to cross the blood–brain barrier (more lipophilic).

Other anticonvulsants: Ongoing therapeutic options can include phenytoin/fosphenytoin and phenobarbital. Phenobarbital may be a good option for seizure prophylaxis as it can be used in the SC route.[7]

Superior Vena Cava Syndrome

SSVC syndrome is usually caused by SVC obstruction (most commonly extra luminal), intraluminal or invasive tumor, or thrombosis. The patient may present with an indolent or more acute symptom profile including dyspnea, facial edema, headache, cough, chest pain, or visual disturbance. There is often a positional element to the symptoms (i.e., sitting up).[8]

Physical examination may reveal facial plethora/cyanosis, proximal vein dilation, and edema to the arm.

Access to definitive diagnostics may be limited in resource-limited environments, thus the diagnosis may be clinical. Chest X-ray and POCUS may assist in clinical decision-making when CT is not available.

Definitive treatment options can be considered, such as stenting, radiotherapy, chemotherapy, and anticoagulation, if possible. Reasonable options for treating a patient with suspected SVC syndrome during a crisis include the following:[9]

• Elevation of the head of the bed
• Symptomatic treatment of dyspnea with low-dose opiates
• Steroid administration (e.g., dexamethasone). This may be sufficient therapy in some patients.
• Diuretics may help to decrease preload.

Dosing details for medications can be found in Chapter 13.

Malignant Spinal Cord Compression

A very commonly missed diagnosis in the face of cancer is malignant spinal cord compression (MSCC). It is a true palliative emergency because if it is not recognized promptly and treated urgently, it leads to significant morbidity, including permanent paralysis, sensory loss, and autonomic dysfunction as well as sphincter loss. Ability to ambulate prior to treatment is a positive prognostic sign, as there is an 80% chance of maintaining this function after treatment.[10] Significant loss of motor function (including walking) before treatment predicts a more dismal rate of recover to walk (approximately 10%).

Commonly associated cancers include breast, lung, prostate, renal, and thyroid. The most common level of compression is the thoracic spine (70%), followed by lumbar and cervical. Multiple levels of compression occur about 30% of the time, thus imaging of the entire spine is strongly recommended.

Pain (dull, sharp, radicular) is the most common presenting feature and most often precedes any neurological deficit (although pain may be rarely absent). On examination, lesions found to be above the L1 level will often demonstrate upper motor neuron signs (hyperreflexia and motor weakness and increased tone), and those lesions below L1 more commonly show lower motor neuron signs (motor weakness, hyporeflexia, and decreased reflexes). Loss of bowel and bladder function is often a late finding and is a poor prognostic indicator.

If MSCC is considered, immediate treatment should be initiated in the form of steroids (e.g., dexamethasone—refer to Chapter 13 for dosing details).

Unfortunately, the diagnostic gold standard is full spinal magnetic resonance imaging (MRI), which is likely not an option during a humanitarian crisis. Plain X-rays are thought not to be useful, though a CT myelogram can be considered if available.[11]

Definitive therapy includes radiotherapy and surgery, if possible. Optimally, MSCC would be an indication for transfer to a referral center.

Ethics of Medical Intervention During an Emergency

In the setting of a humanitarian crisis, the ability to respond to an emergency in a patient with a palliative trajectory may be limited. Often patients with a limited prognosis such as end-stage cancer or organ failure will be subject to triage bias in the face of competing interests (e.g., patients with a reversible medical crisis). Such patients are at risk of suffering in the context of an overwhelmed humanitarian response. The concept of triage in crisis is addressed in detail in Chapter 2.

A key priority would be to make suffering part of triage criteria so that these patients do not go without having their symptom needs addressed. Even if a patient is not expected to survive, quick attention to pain, dyspnea, confusion, nausea, and other distressing symptoms can be easily tackled with low technology options, such as the following:

- Morphine as needed for pain, dyspnea. If available, fentanyl provides rapid onset and is likely a better option for end-stage renal and liver disease, owing to lack of metabolite accumulation.
- Midazolam is often offered for end-stage agitation and delirium, seizures, and dyspnea. One can also utilize infusion for palliative sedation.
- Haldol may be used for agitation and delirium as well as nausea.
- Methotrimeprazine (also known as levomepromazine) is a phenothiazine neuroleptic that may be considered for treating nausea and hyperactive delirium, as well as having some analgesia qualities.

Please refer to Chapter 13 for medication dosing details.

References

1. Hulme B, Wilcox S; Yorkshire Palliative Medicine Clinical Guidelines Group. Guidelines on the management of bleeding for palliative care patients with cancer. 2008. https://www.palliativedrugs.com/download/090331_Final_bleeding_guideline.pdf. Accessed June 29, 2019.

2. Geist MJP, Kessler J, Frankenhauser S, Bardenheuer HJ. Bleeding control in palliative care patients with the help of tranexamic acid. *J Palliat Care*. 2017;32(2) 47–48.

3. Pereira J, Phan T. Management of bleeding in patients with advanced cancer. *Oncologist*. 2004;9(5):561–570.

4. Requarth J. Image-guided palliative care procedures. *Surg Clin North Am*. 2011;91(2):367–402.

5. Ali MS, Sorathia L. Palliative care and interventional pulmonology. *Clin Chest Med*. 2018;39(1):57–64.

6. Leon Ruiz M, Rodriguez Sarasa ML, Sanjuan Rodriguez L, Perez-Nieves MT, Ibanez Estellez F. Guidelines for seizure management in palliative care: proposal for an updated clinical practice model based on a systematic literature review. *Neurolgia*. 2017;34(3):1–33.

7. Mendlik MT, McFarlin J, Kluger BM, Vaughan CL, Phillips JN, Jones CA. Top ten tips palliative care clinicians should know about for patients with neurologic illness. *J Palliat Med*. 2019;22(2):193–198.

8. Staka C, Ying J, Kong FM, Willey CD, Kaminski J, Kim DW. Review of evolving etiologies, implications and treatment strategies for the superior vena cava syndrome. *Springerplus*. 2016;5:229.

9. Portenoy RK, Ahmed E. Cancer pain syndromes. *Hematol Oncol Clin North Am*. 2018;32(3):371–386.

10. Ferrone M, Cheville A, Balboni T, Abrahm J. Update on spinal cord compression for the palliative care clinician. *J Pain Symptom Manage*. 2017;54(3):394–399.

11. Patel DA, Campian JL. Diagnostic and therapeutic strategies for patients with malignant epidural spinal cord compression. *Curr Treat Options Oncol*. 2017;18:53.

Chapter 12

Pediatric Palliative Care in the Context of Humanitarian Crises

Elisha Waldman and Justin N. Baker

Special Pediatric Needs

Children represent a particularly vulnerable and at-risk population in the context of humanitarian crises, especially when it comes to palliative care needs. While many principles of palliative care and symptom management are fairly similar between adults and children, there are a number of important differences. Some conditions seen in children, in particular genetic and metabolic conditions and congenital anomalies, may not be familiar to and readily identifiable by adult practitioners. Additionally, eliciting reports of symptoms and responses to interventions may be challenging, especially in the case of nonverbal children. Occasionally, due to young age or to disease or injury, a child may be unable to speak for him- or herself. In these situations children are at particular risk for symptoms to be underreported and underappreciated and therefore inadequately addressed. Fortunately, medications used are largely the same for adults and children, albeit with some differences in approaches to dosing (as noted later in the chapter and in Chapter 13).

Managing the needs of children presents a unique psychosocial challenge given their place within a family unit and the possibility that the family unit may be absent or damaged. In communicating with children, such as providing anticipatory guidance or assessing goals of care and discussing plans, we typically rely on communication with parents and the larger family structure, especially when children are too young to speak for themselves. In the context of humanitarian crises, the normal family structure may be disrupted (e.g., parent missing or dead) or altogether absent, requiring that special attention be paid to communicating directly with the child.

Children are also at increased risk for psychological and emotional trauma as a result of a crisis; for children who may live for some time (even years) with chronic illness, this sort of trauma increases the risk of long-term morbidity and mortality. Incorporating multidisciplinary support, whenever possible, from psychosocial clinicians such as social workers, psychologists, and chaplains and from other support services such as teachers, art therapists, or child life specialists is critical.

Communication

As noted, primary communication is often with family and guardians and not with children themselves. Whenever possible, children should be directly addressed in an age-appropriate manner. In delivering difficult news, the rule of thumb is generally to "follow the child" and let them tell you what they want to know. Use of play and art can be very helpful when communicating with children. Trusting relationships are also critical to communicating with children, so utilization of clinicians and providers with any prior knowledge of the patient, if available, can be very helpful.

General Approaches to Communicating with Children

- Involve parents and family members whenever possible (infants and younger children may prefer to remain in a family member's arms).
- Remember that children may have been exposed to serious emotional and/or physical trauma. They may now be separated from parents and family, which may heighten a sense of vulnerability. Do your best to remain calm and speak to them in an age-appropriate manner.
- In communicating with children of all ages, be aware of your tone, posture, gestures, and facial expressions. Position yourself at the level of the child so you are speaking eye to eye (not looming over them).
- Communication (and ability to conceptualize death) varies by developmental stage and age. None of these categories are fixed, and, of course, some children may be more advanced than others.
- In general, ask open-ended questions and allow the child and family member, if present, to lead you where they want to go.

General Guidelines for Preferred Communication Styles and Concepts of Death

Infants
- Nonverbal communication
- Tone, volume of speech, gestures, and facial expressions are particularly important at this stage.
- Physical contact such as hugging and rocking may be effective and soothing.
- No concept of death, but aware of separation, which may be disturbing

Age 2–4 Years
- Verbal, prefer concrete questions
- Conceive of death as something reversible (e.g., may still expect deceased family members to return)

Age 4–8 Years
- Still prefer concrete questions, more ability to respond to open-ended questions
- Later in age range idea of death as permanent develops

- Some magical thinking about causes of death (may include assigning blame, e.g., "if I hadn't done that, this wouldn't have happened.")

Age 8–12 Years

- May be more demanding of answers, more able to start engaging in developed conversations
- Concept of personal mortality emerges
- More interest in what happens after death, recognizing its permanence

Age 12 Years and Older

- Ability to understand abstract ideas (including abstract and philosophical ideas around death)
- Able to express full range of emotions

Symptom Management

In general, symptoms encountered and their management resemble that seen in adults.

Some conditions, however, may be less familiar to clinicians more accustomed to adult medicine, including genetic and metabolic conditions and congenital anomalies. These conditions may have been previously undiagnosed, and families may be more or less aware of their extent and meaning. In the context of a crisis, the first priority is determining whether there is any possibility of diagnosing and intervening in a condition. For example, is it at all possible to determine the cause of suspected hydrocephalus or cyanotic heart disease, and is there any ability to intervene? In many, if not most, cases the answer to both may be no, thus the best path is to treat symptomatically, even in the absence of a final diagnosis.

Most distressing symptoms in pediatric palliative care can usually be managed in a stepwise fashion:

- Step 1: Evaluation
- Step 2: Treat underlying causes
- Step 3: Integrative and rehabilitative/supportive therapies
- Step 4: Pharmacological therapy
- Step 5: Re-evaluation at regular intervals and following interventions

Eliciting symptoms and response to interventions may be challenging, especially in a nonverbal child. Often it is incorrectly assumed that children are not experiencing distressing symptoms if they are quiet and don't speak up; silence should not be taken as a sign of absence of pain or disturbing symptoms. Children experiencing extreme pain, especially if it is pain elicited by movement, may appear very quiet and still in an attempt to not provoke painful stimuli; this behavior may be misinterpreted as lack of disturbing symptoms. When children have experienced chronic pain, changes in vital signs like tachycardia may not be accurate indicators of pain. In general, it is safest to take context into account and start with an assumption that a child may be experiencing distress and to treat accordingly. Tools such as the Face, Leg, Activity, Cry, Consolability (FLACC) scale may be useful in evaluating younger or nonverbal children (see Chapter 4).

Especially in situations with a dearth of medications, one should always remember to employ nonpharmacological interventions. Many of these are noted in other symptom-specific chapters in this manual, but in general, these include keeping the child comfortable (warm or cool, depending on conditions) and often just providing human contact; infants in particular often respond simply to being held (though it should be noted that older children who have been exposed to trauma may react adversely to touch, so even this should be approached with caution). Additionally, loss of a sense of security can worsen symptomatology. The concept of "whole pain" should be explored and all aspects of potential suffering attended to, as things such as fear or existential distress may be driving worsening symptomatology.

Medications used for symptom management in pediatrics are similar to those used for adults. The one main difference is that in newborns and infants, because of differences in metabolism, starting doses are generally one-third to half the dose one would use in older children and adults. As noted earlier, symptom burden is often underappreciated, so one should treat liberally, starting low and titrating up to effect, when necessary.

The Actively Dying Child

Symptom management in caring for the actively dying child is largely the same as that of the actively dying adult (taking into account appropriate dose adjustments and communicating in a developmentally appropriate way with the child when possible). The major difference is the critical nature of communicating effectively with parents and family members, if present. Families should receive detailed anticipatory guidance as to what is happening and what they might expect to see. Physical contact with their child should be facilitated when possible. See Chapter 9 for more details.

Chronic Illness

Some pediatric conditions encountered by the clinician providing humanitarian aid may actually be pre-existing chronic conditions, such as cancer, congenital anomalies, and neurodegenerative conditions. Children and their families may or may not be aware of the nature of those conditions, depending on their previous access to healthcare. Because of this, clinicians may be faced with providing new information about a chronic illness, which may be especially difficult in the context of a larger surrounding crisis. Complete diagnostic information may not be available, and prognostication may be difficult, but careful communication to the best of one's ability, to both child and family, is critical. As mentioned earlier, trusting relationships are critical to communicating with children so utilization of clinicians and providers with any prior knowledge of the patient, if available, can be very helpful. Additionally, when considering chronic illness, the question of what longer-term placement and healthcare options might be available must be considered. For example, depending on the crisis, is evacuation to a more developed country a possibility? Placement long term may be a challenging issue, especially if family structure has been disrupted.

Pediatric Medication Dosing

Medications used in pediatric palliative care are largely the same as those used in adult palliative care, with appropriate dose adjustments. In general, when in doubt, pediatric providers recommend going "low and slow," starting with lower doses, especially when dealing with opioids and benzodiazepines, and up-titrating to effect. See Chapter 13 for specific dosing guidelines, and Chapter 9 for a pediatric-specific management algorithm for dying children.

Chapter 13

Essential Medicines

Catherine Habashy, Sarah L. Comolli, and Justin N. Baker

Introduction

The Essential Medicines List (EML) was first developed by the World Health Organization (WHO) in 1977 as a means of promoting equitable access to safe, effective, and low-cost medicines directed at the priority health conditions of a global population.[1] Essential medicines (EM) are a requirement of basic health systems, and access to EM is considered part of the human right to the highest attainable standard of health.[2]

Since its inception, the EML has been revised, expanded, and adapted for specific populations, such as children[3] and patients receiving palliative care.[4] Discrepancies invariably exist between the WHO EML, national EMLs, and recommendations put forth by expert committees and multilateral organizations.[1]

This chapter aims to provide a broad overview of medicines commonly used in palliative care and applicable to the provision of palliative care in humanitarian crises, recognizing that a distinction must often be made between what is optimal, what is essential, and what is readily available.

Access to Essential Medicines in Humanitarian Crises

According to WHO estimates, 80% of the global population lacks access to EM required for the relief of pain and other symptoms.[2] Humanitarian emergencies further impede access to EM and other necessary resources by interrupting critical supply chains.

A list of priority EM for the provision of palliative care in humanitarian crises was highlighted in the 2018 WHO document, *Integrating palliative care and symptom relief into the response to humanitarian emergencies and crises*.[5] While not specific to palliative care in humanitarian crises, additional EMLs have been published by the International Association of Hospice and Palliative Care (IAHPC),[6] the *Lancet* Commission,[7] and Médecins San Frontières (Doctors Without Borders).[8]

Box 13.1 collates the recommendations of these sources and includes additional medicines commonly used by the book's authors and international colleagues in the field along with dosage guidelines.

Essential Medicines in Palliative Care

Box 13.1 Essential Medicines and Dosage Guidelines[9,10]

Acyclovir[§]

Drug Class: Antiviral

Indication: Herpes zoster

Common Formulations: 200 mg, 400 mg, 800 mg tablet; 40 mg/mL oral suspension; 50 mg/mL solution for injection

Route of Administration: PO, IV

Dosing Guidelines:
> *Adult*:
>> *Immunocompetent host*: 800 mg PO 5 times daily
>> *Immunocompromised host*:
>>> Dermatomal: 800 mg PO 5 times daily
>>> Disseminated: 10–15 mg/kg/dose IV q8h
> *Pediatric*:
>> *Immunocompetent host*: 10 mg/kg/dose IV q8h
>> *Immunocompromised (HIV–) host*: 10 mg/kg/dose IV q8h
>> *Immunocompromised (HIV+) host*: 20 mg/kg/dose IV q6h

Comments: Dose, route, and duration vary with indication and immune status; review of indication-specific guidelines is recommended.

Amitriptyline[*†‡§]

Drug Class: Tricyclic antidepressant

Indication: Neuropathic pain, depression (second-line agent)

Common Formulations: 10 mg, 25 mg, 50 mg, 75 mg, 100 mg, 150 mg tablet

Route of Administration: PO

Dosing Guidelines:
- **Neuropathic pain**
  Adult: 10–25 mg PO at bedtime; increase gradually at intervals of ≥1 week; limited benefit beyond doses of 50 mg/day
  Pediatric: 0.1 mg/kg/day at bedtime; increased gradually at intervals of ≥1 week to max dose of 0.5 to 2 mg/kg/day
- **Major depression**
  Adult: 25–50 mg PO at bedtime; increase gradually at intervals of ≥1 week to usual dose of 100–300 mg/day
  Pediatric: Not recommended

Comments: Sedating (nighttime administration recommended); anticholinergic side effects may be dose limiting.

Bisacodyl[*†‡§]

Drug Class: Stimulant laxative

Indication: Constipation

Common Formulations: 5 mg, 10 mg tablet; 10 mg rectal suppository

Route of Administration: PO, PR

Dosing Guidelines:
Adult: 5–15 mg PO once daily as needed
Pediatric:
    3–5 yo: 5 mg PO or PR once daily as needed
    >10 yo: 5–10 mg PO or PR once daily as needed

Carbamazepine[†]

Drug Class: Anticonvulsant

Indication: Neuropathic pain (second- or third-line agent)

Common Formulations: 100 mg, 200 mg tablet; 100 mg/5 mL oral suspension

Route of Administration: PO

Dosing Guidelines:
Adult: 100 mg PO twice daily; increase to 100–200 mg q4–6h (max dose 1200 mg daily)
Pediatric: No guidelines for use in neuropathic pain

Comments: Baseline complete blood count (CBC) should be considered due to rare incidence of aplastic anemia and agranulocytosis; fatal dermatological reactions including toxic epidermal necrolysis (TEN) and Stevens-Johnson syndrome (SJS) may occur.

Chlorpromazine

Drug Class: First-generation (typical) antipsychotic

Indication: Nausea, intractable hiccups

Common Formulations: 10 mg, 25 mg, 50 mg tablet; 25 mg/mL injection

Route of Administration: PO, IV

Dosing Guidelines:
Adult: 10–25 mg q4–6h as needed (nausea); 25–50 mg 3 to 4 times daily (intractable hiccups)
Pediatric (>6 mo): 0.5 mg/kg/dose q6–8h as needed

Comments: Increased mortality observed in elderly patients with dementia-related psychosis who receive antipsychotic agents; use alternate agents when available.

Cimetidine[§]

Drug Class: Histamine antagonist

Indication: Gastric prophylaxis, gastritis, peptic ulcer disease

Common Formulations: 200 mg, 300 mg, 400 mg, 800 mg tablet

Route of Administration: PO

Dosing Guidelines:
Adult: 400 mg at night (prophylaxis); can increase to 300 mg 4 times daily, 400 mg twice daily, or 800 mg at night

Pediatric (≥5 yo and <16 yo): 20–40 mg/kg/day in 3 to 4 divided doses (limited data)

Citalopram[†]

Drug Class: Selective serotonin reuptake inhibitor (SSRI)

Indication: Major depression, generalized anxiety

Common Formulations: 10 mg, 20 mg, 40 mg tablet; 10 mg/5 mL oral solution

Route of Administration: PO

Dosing Guidelines:
Adult: 20 mg once daily, increase at intervals of ≥1 week to max dose of 40 mg/day
Pediatric: Limited data available. Some experts recommend the following:
7–11 yo: 10 mg PO daily, increase by 5 mg/day every 2 weeks (range 20–40 mg/day)
≥12 yo: 20 mg PO daily, increase by 10 mg/day every 2 weeks (range 20–40 mg/day)

Comments: Taper dose when discontinuing to minimize withdrawal symptoms; antidepressants may increase risk of suicidal ideation and behavior in children, adolescents, and young adults.

Dexamethasone[*†‡§]

Drug Class: Corticosteroid

Indication: Nausea, increased intracranial pressure (ICP), bone pain due to metastatic disease

Common Formulations: 0.5 mg, 1 mg, 2 mg, 4 mg tablet; 2 mg/5 mL oral solution; 4 mg/mL solution for injection

Route of Administration: PO, IV, SC

Dosing Guidelines:
Adult: 4–8 mg/day PO/IV/SC (up to 16 mg/day for malignant bowel obstruction or increased intracranial pressure)
Pediatric: 0.15 mg/kg/dose PO/IV q8–12h

Comments: Administer proton pump inhibitor (PPI) or H_2 blocker concurrently; 4 mg/mL solution for injection may be given orally for palatability.

Diazepam[*†‡§]

Drug Class: Benzodiazepine

Indication: Anxiety, agitation, delirium, muscle spasms, seizures

Common Formulations: 2 mg, 5 mg, 10 mg tablet; 5 mg/5 mL oral solution; 5 mg/mL solution for injection

Route of Administration: PO, PR, IV

Dosing Guidelines:

- *Agitation, anxiety, delirium, muscle spasms*
Adult: 2–10 mg PO 2 to 4 times daily
Pediatric: 0.12–0.8 mg/kg/day PO in divided doses q6–8h

- ***Seizures***
    Adult: 0.15–0.2 mg/kg IV (max dose 10 mg), may repeat after 5 minutes
    Pediatric: 0.1–0.3 mg/kg/dose IV (max dose 10 mg), may repeat after
    5 minutes

Comments: IV formulation may be administered rectally if no IV access; use benzodiazepines with caution in the elderly.

Diclofenac[*†‡§]

Drug Class: Nonsteroidal anti-inflammatory drug (NSAID)

Indication: Mild to moderate pain; pain due to inflammatory conditions; adjunctive agent in moderate to severe pain

Common Formulations: 25 mg, 50 mg, 75 mg tablet; 75 mg/3 mL solution for injection

Routes of Administration: PO, IV

Dosing Guidelines:
    Adult: 50 mg PO q8h; 37.5 mg IV q6h (max 150 mg/day)
    Pediatric (1–12 yo): 0.5–3 mg/kg/day, divided 2 to 4 times daily (max 150 mg/day) (limited data, no commercially available liquid formulation)

Comments: Not recommended in renal impairment; consider addition of PPI or H_2 blocker in elderly patients or those at risk for peptic ulcer disease.

Diphenhydramine[*†‡]

Drug Class: Antihistamine

Indication: Pruritus, nausea

Common Formulations: 25 mg tablet; 12.5 mg/5 mL oral solution; 50 mg/mL solution for injection

Route of Administration: PO, IV

Dosing Guidelines:
    Adult: 25–50 mg PO/IV q6–8h as needed
    Pediatric: 1–2 mg/kg/dose PO/IV q6h as needed

Erythromycin

Drug Class: Macrolide antibiotic

Indication: Gastroparesis

Common Formulations: 250 mg tablet; 200 mg/5 mL, 400 mg/5 mL oral suspension

Route of Administration: PO

Dosing Guidelines:
    Adult: 250–500 mg 3 times daily before meals
    Pediatric: 3 mg/kg/dose 4 times daily (max 10 mg/kg or 250 mg)

Comments: Tachyphylaxis may occur with prolonged therapy (>4 weeks).

Fentanyl[†]

Drug Class: Opioid analgesic

Indication: Moderate to severe pain (chronic)

Common Formulations: 12.5 mcg/h, 25 mcg/h, 50 mcg/h, 75 mcg/h, 100 mcg/h patch

Route of Administration: TD

Dosing Guidelines:
Adult: Fentanyl dose should be approximated based on 24-h morphine equivalent
Pediatric: Fentanyl dose should be approximated based on 24-h morphine equivalent

Comments: Providers should be familiar with use; begin only if regular use of PO morphine (or PO morphine equivalent) ≥30 mg daily); time to peak effect is approximately 12 h.

Fluconazole[+‡§]

Drug Class: Antifungal

Indication: Oropharyngeal candidiasis

Common Formulations: 50 mg, 100 mg, 150 mg, 200 mg tablet; 10 mg/mL, 40 mg/mL oral suspension; 2 mg/mL solution for injection

Route of Administration: PO, IV

Dosing Guidelines:
Adult: 200 mg PO/IV on day 1, then 100–200 mg PO/IV daily
Pediatric: 6 mg/kg PO/IV on day 1, then 3–6 mg/kg PO/IV daily

Comments: Dosing of fluconazole varies with indication and immune status; review of indication-specific guidelines is recommended.

Fluoxetine[+‡§]

Drug Class: Selective serotonin reuptake inhibitor (SSRI)

Indication: Major depression, generalized anxiety

Common Formulations: 10 mg, 20 mg tablet; 20 mg/5 mL solution

Route of Administration: PO

Dosing Guidelines:
Adult: 20 mg once daily, increase at intervals of ≥1 week to max dose of 80 mg/day
Pediatric (≥8 yo): 10 to 20 mg/day

Comments: Taper dose when discontinuing to minimize withdrawal symptoms; antidepressants may increase risk of suicidal ideation and behavior in children, adolescents, and young adults.

Furosemide[+‡§]

Drug Class: Loop diuretic

Indication: Pulmonary edema due to heart failure, large-volume ascites due to end-stage liver disease (generally in conjunction with spironolactone)

Common Formulations: 20 mg, 40 mg, 80 mg tablet; 10 mg/mL, 40 mg/5 mL oral solution; 10 mg/mL solution for injection

Route of Administration: PO, IV, SC

Dosing Guidelines:

Adult: 40–80 mg PO q6h; 20–40 mg IV/SC q6h

Pediatric: 2 mg/kg/dose PO q6h, increase in increments of 1–2 mg/kg/dose; 1 mg/kg/dose IV/SC q6h, increase in increments of 1 mg/kg/dose

Comments: Poor bioavailability, particularly in the setting of volume overload; use of diuretics can result in electrolyte abnormalities; furosemide is often administered in conjunction with spironolactone to avoid iatrogenic hypokalemia.

Gabapentin[†]

Drug Class: Anticonvulsant

Indication: Neuropathic pain

Common Formulations: 300 mg, 600 mg, 800 mg tablet; 250 mg/5 mL oral solution

Route of Administration: PO

Dosing Guidelines:

Adult: Initial dose 100–300 mg 1 to 3 times daily; increase to target range of 300 to 1200 mg 3 times daily

Pediatric: Initial dose 10–15 mg/kg/day in 3 divided doses; titrate as tolerated to effective dose (up to 50 mg/kg/day is well tolerated)

Comments: May cause sedation, particularly in combination with opioids; requires slow titration to effective dose; use caution in renal impairment.

Haloperidol[*†‡§]

Drug Class: Typical antipsychotic

Indication: Nausea, agitation, delirium (first-line)

Common Formulations: 0.5 mg, 1 mg, 2 mg, 5 mg, 10 mg, 20 mg tablet; 2 mg/mL oral solution; 5 ml/mL solution for injection

Route of Administration: PO, IV, IM (only when agitation poses safety risk), SC

Dosing Guidelines:

- **Nausea**
  Adult: 0.5–1 mg PO/SC q6h (max 6 mg/day)
  Pediatric (>3 yo): 0.01–0.05 mg/kg/dose PO q8h (limited data)
- **Agitation, delirium**
  Adult: 0.5–5 mg PO/IV 2 to 3 times daily
  Pediatric (3–12 yo): 0.5 mg/day PO in 2 to 3 divided doses; 0.05–0.5 mg/kg/day IV in 3 to 4 divided doses

Comments: Parkinsonian-like syndrome may occur.

Hyoscine butylbromide[*†‡§]

Drug Class: Anticholinergic

Indication: Nausea, visceral pain, oropharyngeal or respiratory secretions

Common Formulations: 10 mg tablet; 20 mg/mL oral solution; 20 mg/mL solution for injection

Route of Administration: PO, IV, SC

Dosing Guidelines:
Adult: 10–20 mg PO/IV/SC 3 to 5 times daily (max 60 mg/day)
Pediatric: Limited data

Comments: Dosage of hyoscine butylbromide and hydrobromide is not equivalent.

Hyoscine hydrobromide

Drug Class: Anticholinergic

Indication: Nausea, visceral pain, oropharyngeal or respiratory secretions, sedation

Common Formulations: 0.4 mg/mL solution for injection

Route of Administration: IV, SC

Dosing Guidelines:
- ***Nausea***
  Adult: 0.6–1 mg IV/SC as needed
  Pediatric: 6 mcg/kg/dose (max 0.3 mg) IV q6–8h as needed
- ***Sedation***
  Adult: 0.3–0.6 mg IV/SC 3 to 4 times daily

Comments: Dosage of hyoscine butylbromide and hydrobromide is not equivalent; central effects only with hydrobromide.

Ibuprofen[*†‡§]

Drug Class: Nonsteroidal anti-inflammatory drug (NSAID)

Indication: Mild to moderate pain; pain due to inflammatory conditions; adjunctive agent in moderate to severe pain.

Common Formulations: 200 mg, 400 mg, 600 mg; 200 mg/5 mL oral suspension

Route of Administration: PO

Dosing Guidelines:
Adult: 200–800 mg (usual dose 400 mg) 3 to 4 times daily (max 3200 mg/day)
Pediatric (>6 mo): 10 mg/kg/dose 4 times daily (max 40 mg/kg/day)

Comments: Not recommended in renal impairment; consider addition of PPI or H_2 blocker in elderly or those at risk for peptic ulcer disease.

Ketamine

Drug Class: Dissociative anesthetic

Indication: Severe pain (subanesthetic dosing)

Common Formulations: 10 mg/mL, 50 mg/mL, 100 mg/mL injection

Route of Administration: IV, intranasal

Dosing Guidelines:
- ***Acute Pain***
  Adult: 0.7 mg/kg intranasal prior to painful procedure[11]
  Pediatric 0.7–1.5 mg/kg intranasal prior to painful procedure[11,12]

- **Chronic Pain**
  Adult: 0.1–0.2 mg/kg/h IV as continuous infusion
  Pediatric: 0.1–0.2 mg/kg/h IV as continuous infusion[13]

Comments: Contraindicated in infants <3 mo due to risk of airway obstruction, laryngospasm, and apnea.

Lactulose[*‡§]

Drug Class: Osmotic laxative

Indication: Constipation

Common Formulations: 10 mg/15 mL oral solution

Route of Administration: PO

Dosing Guidelines:
  Adult: 10–20 g PO daily
  Pediatric: 1–2 g/kg/day in 1 to 2 divided doses

Comments: Can be given as enema; mix with water or normal saline (NS) and use rectal balloon catheter; retain for 30–60 min.

Loperamide[*†‡§]

Drug Class: Antidiarrheal

Indication: Diarrhea

Common Formulations: 2 mg tablet

Route of Administration: PO

Dosing Guidelines:
  Adult: 4 mg, followed by 2 mg after each loose stool
  Pediatric (6–11 yo, 22–43 kg): 2 mg after first loose stool followed by 1 mg after each subsequent loose stool

Comments: Use with caution in patients with suspected infectious colitis.

Lorazepam[*†]

Drug Class: Benzodiazepine

Indication: Nausea (first-line agent for anticipatory nausea), agitation, seizures

Common Formulations: 0.5 mg, 1 mg, 2 mg tablet; 2 mg/mL solution for injection

Route of Administration: PO, SL, IV, SC

Dosing Guidelines:
- **Nausea**
  Adult: 0.5–2 mg PO/IV/SC q6h as needed
  Pediatric: 0.04–0.08 mg/kg/dose PO/IV (max 2 mg) q6h as needed
- **Agitation**
  Adult: 0.02–0.06 mg/kg/dose (max 2 mg) IV/SC q2–6h as needed
  Pediatric: 0.05 mg/kg/dose IV q6h as needed
- **Seizures, status epilepticus**
  Adult: 0.1 mg/kg/dose (max 4 mg) IV, may repeat in 5–10 minutes
  Pediatric: 0.05–0.1 mg/kg (max 4 mg) IV, may repeat in 5–10 minutes

Comments: Use benzodiazepines with caution in the elderly.

Megestrol acetate[†]

Drug Class: Progestin

Indication: Anorexia, cachexia

Common Formulations: 20 mg, 40 mg, 160 mg; 40 mg/mL oral solution

Route of Administration: PO

Dosing Guidelines:
Adult: 40 mg PO 4 times daily
Pediatric: 7.5–10 mg/kg/day in 1 to 2 divided doses (limited data)

Comments: Associated with increased risk of thrombosis.

Meloxicam[†‡]

Drug Class: Nonsteroidal anti-inflammatory drug (NSAID)

Indication: Mild to moderate pain; pain due to inflammatory conditions; adjunctive agent in moderate to severe pain.

Common Formulations: 7.5 mg, 15 mg tablet

Route of Administration: PO

Dosing Guidelines:
Adult: 7.5 mg once daily; may increase to 15 mg once daily
Pediatric (≥2 yo): 0.125 mg/kg daily (max dose 7.5 mg daily)

Comments: Not recommended in renal impairment; consider addition of PPI or H_2 blocker in elderly patients or those at risk for peptic ulcer disease.

Metamizole

Drug Class: Nonopioid analgesic and antipyretic

Indication: Mild to moderate pain, fever

Common Formulations: 500 mg/mL solution for injection

Route of Administration: PO (preferred), IV

Dosing Guidelines:
Adult: 500 mg PO q8h as needed[14]
Pediatric: 10–15 mg/kg/dose PO q6–8h[14]

Comments: Previously removed from many national formularies due to association with fatal agranulocytosis; recent evidence suggests improved safety profile; IV administration is associated with hypotension and bronchospasm.

Methadone[†]

Drug Class: Opioid

Indication: Chronic, moderate to severe pain; mixed nociceptive and neuropathic pain

Common Formulations: 5 mg, 10 mg tablet; 1 mg/mL oral solution

Route of Administration: PO

Dosing Guidelines (opioid naïve):
> *Adult:* 2.5 mg q8h; increase dose by 20–30% every 5–7 days; once stable dose is reached, extend dosing interval to q8–12h
> *Pediatric (>6 mo):* 0.1–0.2 mg/kg/dose q6–8h; increase by 20–30% of total daily dose every 5–7 days; once stable dose is reached, extend dosing interval to q8–12h

Comments: Prescribers should have specialized training in use of methadone; high interpatient variability in elimination half-life exists, and accumulation can occur with repeated dosing; steady-state concentration usually are not attained until 3–5 days after dose change; please see manufacturer's labeling instructions on conversion from other opioids to methadone.

Metoclopramide[*†‡§]

Drug Class: Prokinetic agent

Indication: Gastrointestinal dysmotility, partial bowel obstruction

Common Formulations: 10 mg tablet, 5 mg/5 mL oral solution, 5 mg/mL solution for injection

Route of Administration: PO, IV (SC less preferable)

Dosing Guidelines:
> *Adult:* 10 mg PO/IV q4–6h
> *Pediatric:* 0.0375 mg/kg PO/IV q6h (limited data)

Comments: Contraindicated in complete bowel obstruction; risk of tardive dyskinesia increases with duration of treatment and total cumulative dose; limit use to <12 weeks.

Metronidazole[*‡§]

Drug Class: Antibiotic

Indication: Infectious colitis, topical treatment for open or fungating wounds

Common Formulations: 250 mg, 500 mg tablet

Route of Administration: PO, topical

Dosing Guidelines:
- ***Infectious colitis***:
  > *Adult:* 500–750 mg PO q8h
  > *Pediatric:* 30–50 mg/kg/day PO divided 3 times daily (max 2250 mg/day)
- ***Open or fungating wounds***:
  > Crush tablet and apply topically to open wounds

Midazolam[†]

Drug Class: Benzodiazepine

Indication: Status epilepticus, palliative sedation

Common Formulations: 1 mg/mL, 5 mg/mL injection

Route of Administration: IV, IM, SC, intranasal, buccal

Dosing Guidelines:
- *Seizures*
  Adult: 0.2 mg/kg IM/intranasal (max dose 10 mg), 0.5 mg/kg buccal
  Pediatric: 0.2 mg/kg IM (max dose 6 mg); 0.2 mg/kg intranasal (max dose 10 mg, divide dose between nares); 0.5 mg/kg buccal (max dose 10 mg)
- *Palliative sedation*
  Adult: 0.5–1 mg/h IV/SC; titrate to effect (range 1–20 mg/h)

Comments: Short half-life, generally administered as continuous infusion for sedation; may be administered via IM, intranasal, or buccal route for treatment of seizures.

Mineral oil enema†

Drug Class: Lubricant laxative

Indication: Constipation

Common Formulations: 118 mL enema

Route of Administration: PR

Dosing Guidelines:
  Adult: 118 mL as single dose PR once daily as needed
  Pediatric:
    2 to 11 yo: 30–60 mL PR once daily as needed
    ≥ 12 yo: 60–150 mL PR once daily as needed

Mirtazapine†

Drug Class: Tetracyclic antidepressant

Indication: Major depression, nausea

Common Formulations: 15 mg, 30 mg tablet

Route of Administration: PO

Dosing Guidelines:
  Adult: 15 mg PO at bedtime, increase in intervals ≥1 week (max 45 mg/day)
  Pediatric: Limited data

Comments: Sedation and weight gain are significant side effects; onset of action is faster than with SSRIs; taper dose when discontinuing to minimize withdrawal symptoms.

Morphine*†‡§

Drug Class: Opioid analgesic

Indication: Moderate to severe pain (first-line); dyspnea due to advanced disease or at end of life

Common Formulations: 15 mg, 30 mg tablet; 10 mg/5 mL oral solution; 10 mg/mL solution for injection

Route of Administration: PO, SL, IV, SC

Dosing Guidelines:
  Adult: 5–15 mg PO/SL q4–6h; 2–5 mg IV/SC q2–4h as needed or scheduled
  Pediatric: 0.15–0.3 mg/kg/dose PO/SL q4–6h; 0.05–0.15 mg/kg/dose IV/SC q2–4h as needed or scheduled

Comments: Increase dose by 25–50% if ineffective; respiratory suppression is rare with appropriate titration; constipation is common and may be severe; begin scheduled laxative when starting scheduled opioid.

Naloxone[*‡§]

Drug Class: Opioid antagonist

Indication: Reversal of respiratory depression caused by opioid analgesics

Common Formulations: 0.4 mg/mL, 1 mg/mL solution for injection

Route of Administration: IV, SC

Dosing Guidelines:
   Adult: 0.02–0.2 mg IV/SC as needed
   Pediatric: 0.001–0.005 mg/kg/dose IV as needed

Comments: Opioid-induced respiratory suppression is rare with appropriate initial dosing and titrate; use of naloxone is not recommended for sedation without respiratory depression; administer the lowest dose and titrate slowly to effect; may cause withdrawal or severe pain.

Naproxen[*‡]

Drug Class: Nonsteroidal anti-inflammatory drug (NSAID)

Indication: Mild to moderate pain, pain due to inflammatory conditions; adjunctive agent in moderate to severe pain

Common Formulations: 220 mg, 500 mg tablet; 25 mg/mL oral suspension

Route of Administration: PO

Dosing Guidelines:
   Adult: 250 mg PO q6h or 500 mg PO q12h
   Pediatric (>2 yo): 10 mg/kg/day PO in 2 divided doses (max 15 mg/kg/day)

Comments: Not recommended in renal impairment; consider addition of PPI or H_2 blocker in elderly patients or those at risk for peptic ulcer disease.

Octreotide[†]

Drug Class: Somatostatin analogue

Indication: Malignant bowel obstruction

Common Formulations: 100 mcg/mL, 500 mcg/mL solution for injection

Route of Administration: IV, SC

Dosing Guidelines:
   Adult: 200–900 mcg/day IV/SC in 2 to 3 divided doses
   Pediatric: 1–10 mcg/kg/day IV divided into 1 to 3 doses or administered by continuous infusion (max 1500 mcg/day)

Omeprazole[*‡§]

Drug Class: Proton pump inhibitor (PPI)

Indication: Gastric prophylaxis, gastritis, peptic ulcer disease

Common Formulations: 20 mg tablet; 2.5 mg oral packet; 2 mg/mL oral suspension

Route of Administration: PO

Dosing Guidelines:
Adult: 20–40 mg PO once daily
Pediatric (>1 yo to ≤ 16):
    5–10 kg: 5 mg PO daily
    10–20 kg: 10 mg PO daily
    ≥ 20 kg: 20 mg PO daily

Ondansetron[*‡§]

Drug class: Antiemetic

Indication: Nausea

Common Formulations: 4 mg, 8 mg tablet; 4 mg/5 mL oral solution; 2 mg/mL solution for injection

Route of Administration: PO, IV, SC

Dosing Guidelines:
Adult: 4–8 mg PO/IV/SC q8h as needed or scheduled
Pediatric: 0.15 mg/kg/dose PO/IV q8h or 0.45 mg/kg/dose PO/IV q24h as needed or scheduled

Comments: Headache is a common side effect.

Oxycodone[†]

Drug Class: Opioid analgesic

Indication: Moderate to severe pain

Common Formulations: 5 mg, 10 mg, 15 mg, 20 mg, 30 mg tablet

Route of Administration: PO

Dosing Guidelines:
Adult: 5–15 mg PO q4–6h as needed or scheduled
Pediatric: 0.1 to 0.2 mg/kg/dose (for moderate to severe pain, respectively) PO q4–6 h as needed or scheduled

Comments: Increase dose by 25–50% if ineffective; respiratory suppression is rare with appropriate titration; constipation is common and may be severe; begin scheduled laxative when starting scheduled opioid.

Paracetamol (acetaminophen)[*†‡§]

Drug Class: Analgesic, antipyretic

Indication: Mild to moderate pain; adjunctive agent in moderate to severe pain

Common Formulations: 500 mg tablet; 120 mg/5 mL, 250 mg/5 mL oral solution; 10 mg/mL solution for injection

Route of Administration: PO, PR, IV

Dosing Guidelines:
Adult: 650 mg PO/PR/IV q4–6h (max dose 3–4 gm/day)
Pediatric: 10–15 mg/kg/dose PO/PR/IV q4–6h (max 75 mg/kg/day)

Polyethylene glycol[*‡]

Drug Class: Osmotic laxative

Indication: Constipation

Common Formulation: 17 g/dose powder

Route of Administration: PO

Dosing Guidelines:
Adult: 17 g PO once daily
Pediatric (>6 mo): 0.2–0.8 g/kg/day PO, divided in 1 to 2 doses

Prednisolone†§

Drug Class: Corticosteroid

Indication: Dyspnea secondary to obstructive pulmonary disease; bone pain due to malignant disease; substitute for dexamethasone when not available for nausea, cerebral edema, and increased ICP

Common Formulations: 5 mg tab; 5 mg/5 mL, 10 mg/5 mL, 15 mg/5 mL, 20 mg/5 mL, 25 mg/5 mL oral solution

Route of Administration: PO

Dosing Guidelines:
Adult: 40 mg PO daily
Pediatric: 1–2 mg/kg/day PO, divided in 1 to 2 doses

Comments: Administer PPI or H_2 blocker concurrently.

Prednisone§

Drug Class: Corticosteroid

Indication: Dyspnea secondary to obstructive pulmonary disease; bone pain due to malignant disease; substitute for dexamethasone when not available for nausea, cerebral edema, and increased ICP

Common Formulations: 1 mg, 2.5 mg, 5 mg, 10 mg, 20 mg, 50 mg tablet; 5 mg/5 mL oral solution

Route of Administration: PO

Dosing Guidelines:
Adult: 40 mg PO daily
Pediatric: 1–2 mg/kg/day PO, divided in 1 to 2 doses

Comments: Administer PPI or H_2 blocker concurrently.

Prochlorperazine

Drug Class: Antiemetic, first-generation (typical) antipsychotic

Indication: Nausea

Common Formulations: 5 mg, 10 mg tablet; 5 mg/mL injection

Route of Administration: PO

Dosing Guidelines:
Adult: 5–10 mg 3 to 4 times daily (max 40 mg/day)
Pediatric: Not recommended due to safety profile

Comments: Increased mortality observed in elderly patients with dementia-related psychosis who receive antipsychotic agents.

Promethazine

Drug Class: Antiemetic

Indication: Nausea

Common Formulations: 12.5 mg, 25 mg, 50 mg tablet

Route of Administration: PO

Dosing Guidelines:
Adult: 12.5–25 mg PO q4–6h as needed
Pediatric: (not recommended as first-line agent) 0.25–0.5 mg/kg/dose q4–6h as needed

Comments: Contraindicated in <2 yo due to risk of fatal respiratory depression; IV administration is not recommended due to risk of tissue injury.

Ranitidine

Drug Class: Histamine antagonist

Indication: Gastroesophageal reflux disease (GERD), gastric prophylaxis, gastritis, peptic ulcer disease (PUD)

Common Formulations: 75 mg, 150 mg tablet; 15 mg/mL oral syrup

Route of Administration: PO

Dosing Guidelines:
Adult: 75 mg PO twice daily, can increase to 150 mg PO twice daily
Pediatric: 5–10 mg/kg/day PO divided twice daily (max 300 mg/day)

Senna[+†‡§]

Drug Class: Stimulant laxative

Indication: Constipation

Common Formulations: 8.6 mg tablet, 8.8 mg/5 mL oral solution

Route of Administration: PO

Dosing Guidelines:
Adult: 2 tablets PO (17.2 mg) once daily, can increase to 4 tablets PO twice daily
Pediatric:
2–6 yo: 2.5–3.75 mL PO once daily, can increase to twice daily
6–12 yo: 5–7.5 mL PO once daily, can increase to twice daily

Sertraline[+‡§]

Drug Class: Selective serotonin reuptake inhibitor (SSRI)

Indication: Major depression, generalized anxiety

Common Formulations: 25 mg, 50 mg, 100 mg tablet

Route of Administration: PO

Dosing Guidelines:
Adult: Initial dose 50 mg daily, increase in increments of 25–50 mg weekly to max dose of 200 mg/day
Pediatric (>6 yo): Initial dose 12.5–25 mg once daily, increase in increments of 25–50 mg weekly (mean dose 100 mg/day, max dose 200 mg/day)

Comments: Taper dose when discontinuing to minimize withdrawal symptoms; antidepressants may increase risk of suicidal ideation and behavior in children, adolescents, and young adults.

Sorbitol*‡

Drug Class: Osmotic laxative

Indication: Constipation

Common Formulations: 70% solution

Route of Administration: PO, PR

Dosing Guidelines:
    Adult: 30–45 mL PO as needed; 120 mL PR (diluted to 25–30% solution) as needed
    Pediatric (2–11 yo): 30–60 mL PR (diluted to 25–30% solution) as needed

Spironolactone§

Drug Class: Aldosterone antagonist, potassium-sparing diuretic

Indication: Large-volume ascites in end-stage liver disease, potassium-sparing agent in conjunction with loop diuretics

Common Formulations: 25 mg, 50 mg, 100 mg tab; 5 mg/mL oral suspension

Route of Administration: PO

Dosing Guidelines:
    Adult: 100 mg PO once daily (max 400 mg)
    Pediatric: 1 mg/kg/day PO divided q12–24h

Comments: Furosemide to spironolactone dosing ratio of 40:100 is recommended.

Tramadol†§

Drug Class: Opioid analgesic (weak)

Indication: Moderate to severe pain (second-line agent when standard opioids are not available)

Common Formulations: 50 mg tablet; 10 mg/mL oral solution

Route of Administration: PO

Dosing Guidelines:
    Adult: 50 mg PO q4–6h as needed; may be increased to 50–100 mg q4–6h (max 400 mg/day)
    Pediatric: Limited data to guide use in children. Safety profile is controversial.

Trazodone†

Drug Class: Atypical antidepressant

Indication: Insomnia

Common Formulations: 50 mg, 100 mg tablet

Route of Administration: PO

Dosing Guidelines:
Adult: 50–100 mg at bedtime (max 200 mg)
Pediatric:
18 mo–3 yo: 25 mg at bedtime
>3 yo: 50 mg at bedtime

Zolpidem§

Drug Class: Sedative-hypnotic

Indication: Insomnia

Common Formulations: 5 mg, 10 mg

Route of Administration: PO

Dosing Guidelines:
Adult: 5 mg (women) or 5–10 mg (men) PO immediately before bedtime
Pediatric: Not recommended

Comments: Tolerance may develop rapidly with regular use.

Source of Recommendation: *WHO, *Integrating Palliative Care and Symptom Relief into the Response to Humanitarian Emergencies and Crises*[5]; ‡IAHPC List of Essential Medicines for Palliative Care[6]; †The *Lancet* Commission Report on lack of access to palliative care[7]; §Médecins San Frontières, *Essential Drugs*.[8]

Abbreviation Key: IM, intramuscular; IV, intravenous; mo, months old; PO, by mouth; PR, per rectum; q, every; SC, subcutaneous; SL, sublingual; TD, transdermal; yo, years old.

Essential Equipment in Palliative Care

The following list of essential equipment has been recommended for the provision of palliative care in humanitarian emergencies:
• Pressure-reducing mattress
• Nasogastric drainage and feeding tube
• Urinary catheters
• Opioid lock box
• Flashlight with rechargeable battery (if no access to electricity)
• Adult diapers or plastic and cotton[5]

Subcutaneous Administration of Medication

Intravenous access may be difficult at the end of life. A number of medications may be administered subcutaneously, either intermittently or by continuous infusion (see Box 13.2). Commonly used sites include the anterior abdominal wall, anterior aspect of upper arms, and anterior aspect of thighs.

Subcutaneous medications can be administered using an indwelling winged set (i.e., butterfly) needle when available.[16] A 1 mL saline flush should be administered after single doses or a series of compatible medications. A 1 mL saline flush should be administered between incompatible medications. If compatibility is not known, a 1 mL saline flush should be used in between medications.

> **Box 13.2 Common Medications in Palliative Care that Can Be Administered by Subcutaneous Injection[9,10,16]**
>
> Dexamethasone
> Fentanyl
> Furosemide
> Haloperidol
> Hyoscine butylbromide
> Hyoscine hydrobromide
> Lorazepam
> Metoclopramide (may cause skin irritation)
> Midazolam (may cause skin irritation)
> Morphine
> Naloxone
> Octreotide
> Ondansetron

Subcutaneous catheters should be changed every 7 days, and sooner if redness or induration occur.[16]

References

1. Laing R, Waning B, Gray A, Ford N, 't Hoen E. 25 years of the WHO essential medicines lists: progress and challenges. *Lancet.* 2003;361(9370):1723–1729. doi:10.1016/s0140-6736(03)13375-2

2. Gómez Batiste X, Connor SR (eds.). *Building Integrated Palliative Care Programs and Services.* 2017.

3. World Health Organization. *WHO Model List of Essential Medicines for Children, 5th List.* Geneva: World Health Organization; April 2015. https://www.who.int/medicines/publications/essentialmedicines/en/. Accessed June 30, 2019.

4. World Health Organization. Essential Medicines in Palliative Care Executive Summary. Geneva: World Health Organization; 2017. https://medicalguidelines.msf.org/viewport/MG/en/guidelines-16681097.html. Accessed June 30, 2019.

5. World Health Organization. *Integrating Palliative Care and Symptom Relief into the Response to Humanitarian Emergencies and Crises.* Geneva: World Health Organization; 2018.

6. De Lima L, Doyle D. International Association For Hospice And Palliative Care list of essential medicines for palliative care. *Ann Oncol.* 2006;18(2):395–399. doi:10.1093/annonc/mdl373

7. Knaul FM, et al. Alleviating the access abyss in palliative care and pain relief—an imperative of universal health coverage: the Lancet Commission Report. *Lancet.* 2018;391(10128):1391–1454. doi:10.1016/s0140-6736(17)32513-8

8. Médecins Sans Frontières. *Essential Drugs—Practical Guidelines.* 2018 edition. https://medicalguidelines.msf.org/viewport/MG/en/guidelines-16681097.html. Accessed June 30, 2019.

9. *Uptodate.* 2019. https://www.uptodate.com/home. Accessed April 15, 2019.

10. Wolters Kluver. Clinical Drug Information. Lexicomp, Medi-Span, and Facts & Comparisons. 2019. https://www.wolterskluwercdi.com/. Accessed April 15, 2019.

11. Shrestha R, Pant S, Shrestha A, Batajoo KH, Thapa R, Vaidya S. Intranasal ketamine for the treatment of patients with acute pain in the emergency department. *World J Emerg Med.* 2016;7(1):19. doi:10.5847/wjem.j.1920-8642.2016.01.003

12. Frey TM, Florin TA, Caruso M, Zhang N, Zhang Y, Mittiga MR. Effect of intranasal ketamine vs fentanyl on pain reduction for extremity injuries in children. *JAMA Pediatr.* 2019;173(2):140. doi:10.1001/jamapediatrics.2018.4582

13. Vadivelu N, Schermer E, Kodumudi V, Belani K, Urman RD, Kaye AD. Role of ketamine for analgesia in adults and children. *J Anaesthesiol Clin Pharmacol.* 2016;32(3):298. doi:10.4103/0970-9185.168149

14. Nikolova I, Tencheva J, Voinikov J, Petkova V, Benbasat N, Danchev N. Metamizole: a review profile of a well-known "forgotten" drug. Part I: pharmaceutical and nonclinical profile. *Biotechnology & Biotechnological Equipment.* 2012;26(6):3329–3337. doi:10.5504/bbeq.2012.0089

15. Izhar T. Novalgin in pain and fever. *J Pakistan Med Assoc.* 1999;49(9):226–227.

16. Capital Health. Initiation and administration of medications via an indwelling winged set (subcutaneous butterfly needle). 2007. http://policy.nshealth. ca/Site_Published/dha9/document_render.aspx?documentRender. IdType=6&documentRender.GenericField=&documentRender.Id=27985. Accessed April 15, 2019.

113

Chapter 14

Communicating Bad News

Meaghann S. Weaver and Michaela Ibach

Patients and family members appreciate clear, practical, compassionate, and honest communication delivered in a private setting. Communication of hard news can be considered according to the stages of the conversation, as depicted in Table 14.1.

SPIKES Protocol

The SPIKES protocol offers a practical approach to breaking bad news or sharing sad news (Table 14.2).[1]

Ask-Tell-Ask Method

The Ask-Tell-Ask method serves as an additional communication tool to foster relationship building, a listening presence, and clarification of agenda and understanding when communicating challenging news.

Bonus PRE-ASK: Invest in a pre-ask question to "personalize the patient" and open the conversation with individualized and relational communication. Consider asking a parent to share about a child's personality, asking an adult child what brings their parent comfort or joy, or asking a spouse what strengthens their partner.

ASK: Ask the patient to describe their current understanding of the diagnosis or prognosis or medical issue.

Example questions:

- "To make sure we are on the same page, can you tell me about your medical condition?"
- "What have your other health providers been telling you about your diagnosis or prognosis since the last time we spoke?"

Ask for permission to then "tell" the message of medical update.

TELL: Share the medical news in straightforward language. Craft your "tell" message to take the patient's level of knowledge, emotional state, and degree of education into account.

Stop short of giving a long lecture or huge amounts of detail. Information should be provided in short, digestible chunks with strategic pauses to allow for

Table 14.1. Tangible Tasks for Family Meetings

Time Frame	Recommend	Avoid
Before the meeting	—Preparing academically with the appropriate medical information and review of patient chart and data —Preparing the medical team emotionally	—Rushing into the meeting —Arriving unprepared —Holding the meeting in a public, unexpected place
Opening the meeting	—Introducing everyone present —Inquiring what the family understands —Asking what the family hopes to obtain from the meeting	—Making assumptions about what the family knows —Judging the family's knowledge of prognosis or diagnosis
During the meeting	—Asking about the family's goals —Listening actively —Pausing between statements —Responding appropriately to emotion	—Using medical jargon —Dominating the conversation —Over-speaking or interrupting
Closing the meeting	—Summarizing the meeting content —Exploring the family's understanding —Ensuring ongoing support	—Ending without asking about whether questions and concerns have been addressed —Leaving without committing to a follow-up plan
After the meeting	—Documenting meeting content —Reflecting with self and interdisciplinary team members	—Forgetting self-care and team care or ignoring the emotions associated with the meeting

comfortable silence and processing. A useful rule of thumb is not to give more than three pieces of information at a time. Avoid medical jargon.

ASK: Consider asking the patient to restate what was said in their own words to offer the opportunity to clarify facts and understanding. Provide a chance for the patient or family to ask questions or to request further details.

Tell Me More

A powerful tool in communicating bad news is the phrase "Tell me more, please."[2]

"Tell me more" question tools are as follows:

Tier 1: Could you tell me more about what information you need at this point?

Tier 2: Could you say something about how you are feeling about what we have discussed?

Tier 3: Could you tell me what this means for you?

Table 14.2. SPIKES Protocol

Step	Actionable Approach
1. **S**etting: plan ahead to establish the environment	• Find a quiet, private location if possible and minimize interruptions. • Invite the appropriate people to be present based on necessary staff member inclusion and patient preference on family member presence. • Have tissues nearby. • Ensure enough chairs and sit down with the family.
2. **P**erception: explore what the patient knows already	• "Tell me what you understand about your illness." • "What have the other doctors told you about your illness?" • Look for knowledge and emotional information in the patient's response.
3. **I**nvitation: information-sharing preferences	• "Would it be okay for me to discuss the results of your tests with you now?" • "How do you prefer to discuss medical information in your family?" • "Some people prefer a global picture of what is happening and others like all the details; what do you prefer?"
4. **K**nowledge: give the information	• Give a warning: "I have something serious we need to discuss" or "I'm sorry to say that I have some bad news." • Avoid medical jargon. • Say it simply and stop (e.g., "The tumor has grown—the cancer is getting worse despite our best treatments.")
5. **E**mpathy: respond to emotion	• Wait quietly for the patient. • Use silence therapeutically—silent, supportive presence can be a form of caring well. • "I know this is not what you expected to hear today." • "This is very difficult news."
6. **S**ummary: discuss next steps and follow-up plan	• "We've talked about a lot of things today, please tell me what you understand as the main messages from our meeting." • "Let's set up a follow-up appointment."

Responding to Emotion

Practical strategies for responding to emotion include the following:

• Help the patient to name the emotion through suggestion (never tell a patient how he or she feels): "It sounds like you feel . . . " or "I wonder if you are feeling . . . " or "some people hearing this news would feel. . . ."

• After helping to name the emotion, consider sharing a word of acknowledgment, respect, and empathetic support (e.g., "You're right, this is incredibly [emotion]. I wish things were different and I'm here to support you.").

• Consider involving additional members of the care team, such as the bedside nurse or social worker or behavioral health specialist, to explore different ways to continue to partner with the patient and family.[3]

References

1. Back A, Arnold RM, Baile WF, Tulsky JA, Fryer-Edwards K. Approaching difficult communication tasks in oncology. *CA Cancer J Clin.* 2005;55:164–177.

2. Stone D, Patton B, Heen S. *Difficult Conversations: How to Discuss What Matters Most.* New York: Viking; 2000.

3. Silverman J, Kurtz S, Draper J. *Skills for Communicating with Patients.* Abingdon Oxon, UK: Radcliffe Medical Press; 1998.

Chapter 15

Law and Ethics of End-of-Life Care in Humanitarian Crises

Natasha Yacoub,* Lisa Schwartz, and Kevin Bezanson

Introduction

Patients are often unable to access the end-of-life assistance they need during humanitarian crises. Where humanitarian access may be limited and resources finite, complex ethical issues arise for humanitarian actors in prioritizing palliative care. Saving lives may take precedence over medical care for individuals who cannot be cured or support for their families. However, this also raises serious ethical and legal questions for humanitarian actors. This chapter explores the right of patients to palliative care during emergencies, whether owing to conflict or natural disaster. It argues that there is a legal obligation, primarily of governments, to provide access to palliative care to relieve suffering and respect human dignity in these scenarios, and that the ethics of humanitarian action demands it.

In the context of end-of-life care in humanitarian crises, ethical and legal concerns draw from an important distinction between what palliative care is and what it is *not*. Palliative care is *not* abandoning patients to "no care or treatment," nor is it intentionally ending a patient's life (euthanasia). In reality, palliative care is the opposite of each of these. Rather, it is actively caring for people for whom curative treatment is no longer viable, and it concerns non-abandonment, comfort measures, and attention to psychosocial issues. Moreover, it is intended to be patient centered and family engaged.

The Law

In designing humanitarian interventions, there is a sound legal basis for integrating palliative care into a response targeting multiple rights.

International Human Rights Law

Definition

International human rights law applies in all humanitarian crises, with limited exceptions in a state of emergency. It is often reflected in regional and national laws. This area of law enables advocacy for the inclusion of palliative care in

* The views expressed herein are those of the author and do not necessarily reflect the views of the United Nations.

humanitarian settings; sets out the obligations of state and non-state actors; and provides the framework to document and seek legal recourse for violations of palliative care rights. The foundation of international human rights law, the International Bill of Rights, is the Universal Declaration of Human Rights 1948 (UDHR) as well as two binding treaties, the International Covenant on Civil and Political Rights 1966 (ICCPR)[1] and International Covenant on Economic, Social and Cultural Rights 1966 (ICESCR),[2] signed by almost all states.

Right to Health

Article 12.1 of the ICESCR[2] requires that governments "recognise the right of everyone to the enjoyment of the highest attainable standard of physical and mental health." This right can be interpreted to include a right of patients to receive palliative care as well as an obligation of governments to provide this care.[3] Acknowledging the difficulties of resource-poor nations, the law requires that the right is progressively realized. However, certain aspects are compulsory, including access to minimum essential food, basic shelter, housing, and sanitation; an adequate supply of safe and potable water; and the provision of essential drugs.[4] The essential drugs, defined under the World Health Organization (WHO) Action Program on Essential Drugs, includes medications for common symptoms used in palliative care provision.[5] (Please see Chapter 13 for essential medications and dosing.)

Special Needs

The right to health under international law requires that access to healthcare, which may include palliative care, should be provided during humanitarian crises for groups of people in a non-discriminatory manner and with particular attention to individuals with special needs, including:

- Ethnic minorities (Article 5(e)(iv) of the International Convention on the Elimination of All Forms of Racial Discrimination, 1965)
- Women (Articles 11(1)(f), 12, and 14(2)(b) Convention on the Elimination of All Forms of Discrimination against Women, 1979)
- Children (Article 24 of the Convention on the Rights of the Child, 1989)
- Persons with disabilities (Article 25 of the Convention on the Rights of Persons with Disabilities, 2006)

Prohibition of Torture and Cruel, Inhuman, and Degrading Treatment

Article 7.1 of the ICCPR[1] states that "no one shall be subjected to torture or to cruel, inhuman or degrading treatment or punishment . . . ." The denial by a government of palliative care may comprise cruel and inhuman treatment or even torture if the elements of the law are met. An example of a breach of this law could be the prohibition by a state of the use of opioids for medical purposes.[3]

Cultural Relativism

A common challenge in the provision of palliative care in humanitarian settings is the cultural and religious beliefs about death and dying that may inhibit services such as pain relief or psychological interventions. While humanitarians have a duty to understand and respect local customs and beliefs, culture cannot override fundamental human rights.[6] Respect for human dignity is a common principle of international human rights law that should include the right to die in dignity, recognizing the cultural differences in how dignity is defined.

Remedies

Violations of international human rights law are usually overseen by independent human rights monitors, including non-governmental organizations (NGOs). The United Nations has rapporteurs on particular rights who prepare specialized reports. The legal breaches will be raised with the government concerned, either confidentially or through public reporting. In addition, international human rights treaties have periodic reporting requirements, whereby states report on compliance with the law to a treaty body. Civil society actors may raise concerns about a lack of palliative care to the treaty body through a confidential or public communication with this treaty body. Moreover, there is a procedure to make complaints under some international human rights treaties to specialized bodies, but the recommendations are non-compellable. If international human rights norms are incorporated into regional and domestic laws, then binding decisions may be available through regional or domestic courts.

International Humanitarian Law

Definition

International humanitarian law (IHL), or the law of war, applies during international and non-international armed conflict. It binds both states and parties to a conflict. The principle IHL texts are the four Geneva Conventions of August 12, 1949 and their two Additional Protocols of 1977 relating to the protection of victims in armed conflict.[7] These instruments serve to limit the effects of war by protecting persons who are no longer participating in hostilities, including wounded or sick military and naval personnel and prisoners of war; protecting civilians, including health workers; and restricting the means and methods of warfare. The instruments are principally overseen by the International Committee of the Red Cross (ICRC).[7]

Access to Healthcare

IHL complements international human rights law. It provides specific rules protecting access to healthcare during conflict, which can be interpreted to include end-of-life assistance. For example, Article 12 of the Geneva Convention for the Amelioration of the Condition of the Wounded and Sick in Armed Forces in the Field 1949 requires that the parties to a conflict protect wounded and sick persons from ill treatment, which includes a prohibition on torture. It requires that they they shall not wilfully be left without medical assistance and care. Depriving the sick and wounded of palliative care could be interpreted to violate this provision. The most significant IHL treaties relating to healthcare provision in emergencies are summarized in: https://www.icrc.org/en/document/respecting-and-protecting-health-care-armed-conflicts-and-situations-not-covered.

Remedies for Violations

The ICRC monitors humanitarian crises situations and communicates confidentially with governments and armed actors to remedy breaches of IHL. Where stronger measures are required, there may be diplomatic pressure on the state or armed actors by intergovernmental organizations or interested states. For very serious breaches of the law, criminal justice through specialized tribunals or the International Criminal Court may be available.

Other Laws Applicable in Humanitarian Emergencies

Relevant areas of international law, many reflected in regional and national laws, include refugee law, privileges and immunities law, customs law, and transport law. Duty-of-care obligations may arise under tort law in many national jurisdictions.[8] For more information, see: https://ifrc-media.org/interactive/wp-content/uploads/2015/12/FP-brochure-2015.pdf.

Ethics

Key Ethical Approaches

The key ethical issues guiding palliative care in humanitarian responses may be viewed from a *principlist approach*, namely based on bioethical principles of autonomy, beneficence, nonmaleficence, and justice, or *virtue ethics approach*, applying the principles of virtuous health professionals.[3] The key principles have been described by the WHO as[6]:

- Respect for persons—dignity and human rights are respected, patients have access to information, confidentiality is respected.
- Nonmaleficence—do no harm.
- Beneficence—work for the good of patients and protect them from harm; exercise good judgement in situations where the good of the patient or family conflicts with public health concerns (e.g., restrictions on burial rituals during infectious disease outbreak).
- Justice—equal medical treatment is provided for patients with similar conditions or symptoms, not restricting patient autonomy except to protect public health.[8]
- Solidarity—communities stand together to face common threats and overcome pathogenic inequalities.
- Non-abandonment—no person in need of medical care should be abandoned, ignored, or neglected, and expectant patients much be provided with palliative care and symptom control as essential parts of all humanitarian crises.
- Double effect—an action with a possible good effect and possible bad effects is morally permitted if the action if not immoral, is undertaken with the intention of achieving the possible good effect, does not bring about the possible good effect by means of a possible bad effect, and is undertaken for a proportionately grave reason.
- Ethics and culture—humanitarian actors must seek to understand local ethical norms and adapt them to a patient's religious, cultural, and personal values, noting that culture does not override human rights.

If a conflict between ethical principles arises, the WHO proposes that the ways to resolve these include seeking input from those affected, ensuring two-way communication with all affected people, transparency in explaining decisions, providing a mechanism to challenge decisions, ensuring consistency in allocation, and ensuring that palliative care is accessible for patients who cannot be saved with existing resources.[6]

Humanitarian Principles

Authors, such as Hugo Slim,[9] propose that the first four of the Seven Humanitarian Principles[10] help to define humanitarianism.[9] Taken together, these four principles support an ethical imperative to provide palliative care in crisis situations:

1. Humanity—preventing and alleviating suffering wherever it is found, protecting life and health, ensuring respect for the human being

2. Impartiality—non-discrimination in delivering assistance, endeavoring only to relieve suffering and giving priority to the most urgent cases

3. Neutrality—taking no sides in hostilities

4. Independence—maintaining autonomy so as to be able to act in accordance with the other principles

Thus, the Humanitarian Principles can be understood to require the humane treatment of people who are unable to be cured or whose lives cannot be saved. The principles of humanity and impartiality in particular mean that "all patients receive care and should never be abandoned for any reason, even if they are dying."[6]

Humanitarian actors may also be bound by codes of conduct, which may be enforceable by law.

Obstacles and Moral Experiences

Obstacles

In humanitarian healthcare settings, numerous obstacles to provision of palliative care have been identified. Nevertheless, as Smith and Aloudat[11] have pointed out, there is no need for a false dichotomy between palliative interventions and what humanitarian healthcare has to offer. On the contrary, palliative care can easily harmonize with a stated principle of humanitarian action: to help ease suffering.[11,12–16]

The following obstacles to palliative care in humanitarian settings have been identified[17]:

1. Ethos: the rush to rescue and the emphasis on saving as many lives as possible sometimes leads to feelings of complicity when only end-of-life care can be provided.

2. Priorities: there is an explicit need for triage in many circumstances and ensuing dilemmas about how limited time and resources should best be allocated.

3. Funder expectations: saving lives is believed to be a higher priority and the essence of public engagement for funders, rather than providing palliation for those whose lives cannot be saved.

4. Lack of expertise, training, and guidance for field practitioners to situate palliative care in crisis settings: sometimes this leads to either abandonment

or futile invasive interventions for patients who will only experience them as burdensome and not beneficial.

5. Poor access to adequate pain medications: this can be due to scarcity, or more often to these medications not being authorized or legally obtainable inside an affected country.

6. Apprehension about cultural specificity: understanding how to deliver culturally appropriate care is complicated and will take time and engagement to accomplish.

7. Lack of shared language: about palliation, end-of-life care, and other concepts can lead to misunderstandings and breakdowns in trust among providers and within organizations.

8. Worries about security risks: these are associated with a) being misperceived as providing no care or actively ending lives, and b) concerns about theft of scarce, potentially valuable, pain medications such as opiates.

9. Host community relationships: this is related to cultural sensitivity, but also that inequities may arise in the health system does not, or is unable to provide palliative care services, while an NGO offers it only to the population it is designated to serve, such as refugees. It is also important to recognize that in crisis settings, local healthcare providers and volunteers may be experiencing their own trauma and bereavement.

10. Continuity of care: continuity is a special concern in fragile states or when a field program is intended to be short term. Patients started on palliative care may be unable to access it when the NGO is out of range.

This list may not be exhaustive, but it represent the concerns shared by field practitioners in an empirical study.[17]

Moral Experiences

Confronting the obstacles in the course of disaster relief or in conflict settings can lead to moral distress, where a sense of wanting to do what is best for the patient or community is thwarted by the realities of the context. An examination of the moral experiences of humanitarian healthcare providers providing care for patients with life-limiting illness indicates that values of compassion and justice are at the heart of their efforts.[17] While healthcare providers recognize their duty of care to all patients, they wrestle with being able to manage priorities fairly within emergency settings made worse by scarce resources, leading to the perception that there is no time or capacity for patients with life-limiting illness. Healthcare providers in humanitarian settings identify inequities where patients are excluded from accessing care when there is little availability of healthcare providers trained in palliative approaches to healthcare and/or where internal or external policies limit or exclude access to essential medicines for adequate pain and symptom management. This unfairness has led many to describe frustrations, moral and psychological distress, and residue eventually leading to burnout.[18]

An additional and significant experience is one of the "wounded healer," recognizing that first responders in humanitarian crises are most likely to be people who are members of the effected population. Findings by Yantzi et al.[19] indicate that this will mean that care providers may themselves be injured, traumatized, and managing shock and loss while trying to help others through the same experiences. Those who follow on the scene need to be attentive to the realities and limitations involved, while also respecting the dignity, autonomy, and sovereignty of the first responders in a crisis. These conditions may make it easier or harder for some to accept the limitations of treatment and offer palliative care.

Evidence indicates humanitarian actors are committed to mutual recognition of humanity. They draw on compassion for the people they encounter, provoking a strong desire to meet patients on an equal footing in order to preserve the dignity of patients while they are dying, and to provide palliative care where needed if at all possible.

Recommendations

In any humanitarian setting, some patients will die because of the event, such as disaster, conflict, outbreak of disease, while others will have been dying and in need of palliation even before the event. The professional duty of care extends to all patients, not just those whose lives can be saved or extended. Leaving a dying patient with no care is abandonment and a breach of fiduciary duty. Palliative care has been identified as a right.[3,7,20,21] It is consistent with the commitment of humanitarian actors to attend to those in need and ease suffering. Consequently, palliative care should be integrated into humanitarian response efforts and not be treated as an added option or an unnecessary luxury that distracts from the "real" work of humanitarian response. The following should therefore be considered:

- Training and guidance for field healthcare providers, whether local or expatriate[22,23]
- Fair triage practices that recognize the needs of the dying without triaging-out patients who can benefit from palliative care[17]
- Better understanding of the needs of patients and families with respect to culturally relevant palliative treatment
- Availability of a kit of palliative care resources, including appropriate pain management treatments[8]
- Recognition that the principles and practices of palliative care can extend across the illness trajectory and improve treatment of many other patients
- Acknowledgment that palliative interventions need not be resource intensive. They can include many interventions, from surgery and medicines, to simply arranging for the patient to contact a family member they have be separated from because of the crisis, or finding a volunteer to sit by a patient, hold a hand, and listen to their stories[12,15]
- Inclusion of palliative care in humanitarian response guidance, such as the *Sphere Standards*[24]
- Research is needed to provide data that can improve understanding of the need for palliative care and its impact in humanitarian settings.[11,14,22]

Healthcare providers indicate feeling moral distress at the absence of palliative interventions and guidance. Such interventions will help provide more appropriate and compassionate care for patients living with life-limiting illness or injury and help support families through care and bereavement. An expanded ethos of humanitarian care that integrates palliative approaches will benefit patients, families, and care providers. There is both an ethical and legal imperative to do so.

References

1. UN General Assembly. *International Covenant on Civil and Political Rights.* December 16, 1966. United Nations Treaty Series, Vol. 999, p. 171. https://www.ohchr.org/en/professionalinterest/pages/ccpr.aspx. Accessed June 30, 2019.

2. UN General Assembly. *International Covenant on Economic, Social and Cultural Rights.* December 16, 1966. United Nations Treaty Series, Vol. 993, p. 3. https://www.ohchr.org/en/professionalinterest/pages/cescr.aspx.https://www.ohchr.org/EN/Issues/Education/Training/Compilation/Pages/e)GeneralCommentNo14Therighttothehighestattainablestandardofhealth(article12)(2000).aspx. Accessed June 30, 2019.

3. Brennan F, Gwyther L, Harding R. Palliative Care as a Human Right. Open Society Institute, Law and Health Initiative on Palliative Care and Human Rights; January 2008. https://www.opensocietyfoundations.org/publications/palliative-care-human-right. Accessed June 30, 2019.

4. Office of the High Commissioner for Human Rights. UN Committee on Economic, Social and Cultural Rights (CESCR), General Comment No. 14: The Right to the Highest Attainable Standard of Health (Art. 12). E/C.12/2000/4. August 11, 2000. https://www.refworld.org/pdfid/4538838d0.pdf. Accessed June 30, 2019.

5. World Health Organization (WHO). *WHO Model List of Essential Medicines.* 20th ed. Geneva: World Health Organization; 2017. https://apps.who.int/iris/bitstream/handle/10665/273826/EML-20-eng.pdf?ua=1. Accessed June 30, 2019.

6. World Health Organization (WHO). *Integrating Palliative Care and Symptom Relief into Responses to Humanitarian Emergencies and Crises: A WHO Guide.* Geneva: World Health Organization; 2018. Licence: CC BY-NC-SA 3.0 IGO. https://apps.who.int/iris/handle/10665/274565. Accessed June 30, 2019.

7. International Committee of the Red Cross (ICRC) Advisory Service on International Humanitarian Law. Respecting and Protecting Health Care in Armed Conflict and Situations Not Covered by International Humanitarian Law. Geneva: ICRC; 2012. https://www.icrc.org/en/document/respecting-and-protecting-health-care-armed-conflicts-and-situations-not-covered. Accessed June 30, 2019.

8. Nortjé N, Gwyther L, Kleinschmidt A, Ezer T. Ethical issues. In: *Legal Aspects of Palliative Care.* Cape Town, South Africa: Hospice Palliative Care Association of South Africa and Open Society Institute; 2009. www.hospicepalliativecaresa.co.za/legal resources. Accessed June 30, 2019.

9. Slim H. *Humanitarian Ethics: A Guide to the Morality of Aid in War and Disaster.* London: C. Hurst & Co. Publishers Ltd; 2012.

10. International Federation of Red Cross and Red Crescent Societies (IFRC), International Committee of the Red Cross (ICRC). *The Fundamental Principles of the International Red Cross and Red Crescent Movement: Ethics and Tools for Humanitarian Action.* Geneva: IFRC and ICRC; 2015.

11. Smith J, Aloudat T. Palliative care in humanitarian medicine. *Palliat Med.* 2017;31:99–101. https://doi.org/10.1177/0269216316686258

12. Frahm KA, Brown LM, Gibson M. The importance of end-of-life care in nursing home settings is not diminished by a disaster. *Omega (Westport)*. 2011;64:143–155.

13. Marston J, Lima LD, Powell RA. Palliative care in complex humanitarian crisis responses. *Lancet.* 2015;386(10007):1940. https://doi.org/10.1016/S01406736(15)00825-9

14. Powell RA, Schwartz L, Nouvet E, et al. Palliative care in humanitarian crises: always something to offer. *Lancet* 2017;389:1498–1499. https://doi.org/10.1016/S0140-6736(17)30978-9

15. Rosoff PM. Should palliative care be a necessity or a luxury during an overwhelming health catastrophe? *J Clin Ethics.* 2010;21:312–320.

16. Rosoff PM. Caring for the suffering: meeting the Ebola crisis responsibly. *Am J Bioeth.* 2015;15:26–32. https://doi.org/10.1080/15265161.2015.1010995

17. Hunt M, Chénier A, Bezanson K, et al. Moral experiences of humanitarian health professionals caring for patients who are dying or likely to die in a humanitarian crisis. *J Int Humanit Action.* 2018;3(1):12.

18. Webster GC, Baylis FE. Moral residue. In: Rubin SB, Zoloth L, eds. *Margin of Error: The Ethics of Mistakes in the Practice of Medicine.* Hagerstown, PA: University Publishing Group; 2000:217–230.

19. Yantzi R, et al. Nothing in the world can serve those people like palliative care: qualitative analysis of refugee and provider experiences in Jordan, Rwanda, and Bangladesh. Presentation at MSF Scientific Days; London; May 8–10, 2019.

20. Fowler-Kerry S, Cunningham C. Thinking about the effects of a natural disaster on existing palliative needs. *Int J Palliat Nurs.* 2013;16:255. https://doi.org/10.12968/ijpn.2010.16.5.48147

21. Médecin San Frontières (MSF). Adapting our practices to respect dignity. 2009. http://www.msf.ca/en/article/adapting-our-practices-respect-dignity. Accessed February 16, 2017.

22. Matzo M, Wilkinson A, Lynn J, Gatto M, Phillips S. Palliative care considerations in mass casualty events with scarce resources. *Biosecur Bioterror.* 2009;7:199–210. https://doi.org/10.1089/bsp.2009.0017

23. Nouvet E, Sivaram M, Bezanson K, et al. Palliative care in humanitarian crises: a review of the literature. *J Int Humanitar Action.* 2018;3(1):5.

24. Sphere Association. *The Sphere Handbook: Humanitarian Charter and Minimum Standards in Humanitarian Response.* 4th ed. Geneva: Sphere Association; 2018. https://www.spherestandards.org/handbook. Accessed June 30, 2019.

Chapter 16

Cultural, Psychological, and Spiritual Dimensions of Palliative Care in Humanitarian Crises

Peter Yuichi Clark, Denah M. Joseph, and Jessi Humphreys

Introduction

In focusing on the psychosocial and spiritual needs of patients, families and communities, we are guided by a trauma-informed approach. Trauma is defined as "an event or series of events . . . that is experienced as physically or emotionally harmful or life threatening and has the potential to have lasting adverse effects on mental, physical, social, emotional, or spiritual well-being."[1] Clinicians begin by attending to people's survival needs for acute medical care, food, water, shelter, and security, including symptom management. Only when those are addressed can aid workers attend to the other dimensions of people's experience. Employing best practices, aid organizations would ideally deploy trained colleagues in psychosocial and spiritual support and collaborate with local experts to meet people's multidimensional needs.

Applying Cultural Humility to Unconscious Beliefs and Biases

There is no way to separate a humanitarian crisis from the cultural context in which it occurs. Unconscious and unavoidable cultural assumptions govern how we see the world and shape how we offer care. These beliefs include how we view suffering, death, and dying; how the circumstances surrounding a death affect grief and bereavement; how people construct meaning from their losses; and whether the decision-making model is individual or collectivist.[2,3] As a foundational principle, we assert that cultural self-awareness, cultural humility,[4] and cultural curiosity[5] are essential to providing effective care, whether in the clinic or in a disaster zone.

Core Areas of Concern for Culturally Effective Palliative Care

The most significant contributor to culturally effective palliative care in humanitarian crises is communication. During a crisis it may be challenging to establish trust within the context of great emergency. Following are some common cultural conundrums in humanitarian crises and methods to approach them with humility.

• *Nonverbal communication*: Observe other patients and providers to assess how they respond to vocalization, eye contact, physical contact, gestures, and body language.

• *Decision-making*: Ask individuals how they wish to be involved in decision-making. They may wish to share this role with family, religious leaders, or other community stakeholders.

• *Discussing death, dying, and prognosis*: Ask how individuals or families would like illness discussed; honor preferences for information; address hopes and worries (e.g., "We are also hoping for X, and we worry about Y.").

• *Cultural differences in physical examinations*: Whenever possible, honor cultural preferences for gender of provider for intimate examinations; preserve privacy; cover sensitive body areas, genitals, hair, and face; acknowledge limitations in emergencies.

• *Cultural views of diagnosis and medications*: Explore cultural narratives for diseases, diagnoses, treatments, and the role of healthcare providers; align with beliefs and integrate Western medical interventions with existing practices as feasible.

• *End-of-life rituals and burial practices*: Ask questions; express curiosity and the desire to care for loved ones appropriately. Concerns may include who can touch the body, confessional deathbed prayers, funerary practices, and burial clothing.

• *Safety in funerary and burial practices*: Work directly with community members to ensure both culturally respectful and medically safe compromises when practices may pose a health or infectious concern.

• *Cultural perspectives on suffering*: Apply curiosity and humility without judgment in acknowledging the cultural continuum of grief from reserved to verbally and physically overt.

Mapping the Psychosocial and Spiritual Terrain of Palliative Care in Humanitarian Crises

Common psychosocial and spiritual responses include the following:
• Dysregulated emotional behavior such as rage, terror, and profound grief
• Questioning why one has survived when others have not
• Losing coherence or meaning in one's world
• Losing one's future dreams and hopes

- Confronting one's fragility and mortality
- Fight, flight, and freeze reactions; diminished cognitive processing
- Activation of historical trauma, intrusive thoughts or images

Individuals' vulnerability in the face of crises will vary depending on what coping strategies and supports they have available, their access to safety after a crisis, and the meaning a person attributes to the event. In a protracted humanitarian crisis such as multiyear conflicts, ongoing human rights abuses, and destruction of entire communities, the psychological sequelae may be far more difficult to address and resolve, given the continued trauma.

Factors that can exacerbate psychological morbidity include the following[6]:

- High perceived threat to life, loss of control over outcomes, and an inability to predict whether the threat is ongoing, reoccurring, or contained
- Extensive personal loss—for example, family members, home, safety, functional capacities, usual roles
- Crisis is human-caused (e.g., terrorism, massacre), sudden, shocking, and associated with massive injuries and loss of life
- People are exposed to grotesque circumstances or corpses, especially of children
- Extensive loss of the social and communal safety net

Protective Factors in Stress Resilience and Recovery

Not everyone exposed to traumatic experiences goes on to display long-term psychological morbidity. Rather, it is estimated that approximately 75% of a group enduring a humanitarian crisis display what is termed "psychosocial resilience."[7,8] The remaining 25% run a significant risk of developing psychological distress that does not resolve. It is crucial to direct scarce mental health resources toward those patients who manifest the most severe symptoms.[9]

Psychological First Aid (PFA)

There is growing empirical evidence to support interventional practices and programs in the immediate and mid-term periods following disaster and mass violence. The principles undergirding such interventions are to promote a sense of safety, calm, self- and collective efficacy, connectedness, and hope.[10]

At the time of the actual crisis, *if* it is time limited, "psychological first aid" (PFA) has emerged as a response strategy endorsed by the World Health Organization. Core actions of PFA include the following[9,11]:

- ***Contact and engagement***: Approach survivors who require assistance in a nonintrusive, compassionate, and helpful manner.
- ***Safety and comfort***: Ensure immediate and ongoing safety and attend to physical and emotional comfort needs.
- ***Stabilization:*** Calm emotionally overwhelmed or disoriented survivors, and help them to become better oriented to their surroundings.

- **Information gathering**: Listen to people's stories and identify immediate needs and concerns so as to customize PFA interventions.
- **Connection with social supports**: Establish contact with support persons including family members, friends, and community organizations, agencies, and networks.
- **Information on coping**: Provide information about stress reactions and coping. Normalize emotional responses (e.g., shock, numbing, and/or intense feelings) and the adjustment process (e.g., there is no one "right" way to respond; there is no one "right" timeline for recovery).

Grief and Bereavement During Humanitarian Crises

Because of the high probability of multiple losses in crises, it is helpful to assess which are most pronounced for those one is serving, in order to triage care. Loss can appear in any of the following domains: loss of identity and customary roles, loss of bodily functions, loss of relationships, and material loss. The process of grief and bereavement is a long-term task with an individually and culturally variable timeline. Experts in the field have identified tasks of grief including accepting the reality of the loss, experiencing the emotional pain of grief, and finding an enduring connection with the deceased.[12]

Special Circumstances of Grief: Disappearance of Loved Ones and Uncertainty

Humanitarian crises can result in unique forms of loss, including the disappearance of loved ones and prolonged uncertainty. Disappearance is one of the most challenging losses to process because of its ambiguity,[13] as victims repeatedly vacillate between hope and despair. Losing individuals complicates decision-making, especially for children who would otherwise turn to those individuals for assistance. If the bodies of loved ones cannot be found or identified, certain rituals meant to honor the deceased and affirm a connection between the living and the dead—such as cleansing the body or keeping vigil—are thwarted. Even when the deceased's body is located, preferred multiday funerary rituals may not be feasible given displaced communities.

Spiritual Care in the Midst of Humanitarian Crises

Spiritual care practices in palliative care include helping individuals face and overcome fears and find hope and meaning; attending to existential suffering; addressing feelings of punishment, guilt, unfairness, and remorse; assisting when people need to confess or reconcile; and offering grief support and death preparation assistance. All of these interventions can be facilitated by a skilled listener expressing *human kindness and compassion* as a form of first aid. *Being available for connection, demonstrating acceptance, caring, and concern, with respect and attention to dignity, is the primary spiritual intervention in humanitarian crises.* Studies involving people affected by Louisiana floods in 2016,[14] Hurricanes Katrina and Rita in 2005, the 2010 Deepwater Horizon oil spill,[15] and a 4-year drought in Botswana[16] indicate that perceived spiritual support promotes adaptation responses and can have a protective effect on post-disaster resilience.[17]

For aid organizations to enact best practices in providing comprehensive care, we recommend integrating spiritual care into the long-term strategy of the organization. To this end, it is critical to advocate for spiritual specialists within humanitarian organizations, as well as to partner with local spiritual leaders and faith-specific liaisons.[18]

As a disaster spiritual caregiver, there are several principles of SFA that can help guide specific responses[19]:

- **Stabilization and introduction**: Build rapport and allow for assessment.
- **Acknowledgment**: Listen actively to the person in crisis.
- **Facilitating understanding**: Validate and normalize survivors' experiences by allowing them to express their reactions. Offer basic information about stress.
- **Encouraging adaptive coping**: Identify past positive effective coping strategies for survivors and promote their use.
- **Referral**: Serve as a "bridge" to resources; help to access local community spiritual and religious leaders and religious rituals. In response to hearing, "Why did God allow this to happen?" you might respond, "You're asking a very profound question. I think you might benefit from speaking with someone who can help you explore what is happening. Would you like me to arrange for that person to visit you?"

Disasters and other humanitarian crises compel us to confront forces that are beyond our mastery. They accentuate our fragility, mortality, and smallness in uncomfortable and distressing ways. What is asked of us is to stand with survivors in mutual vulnerability and authentically convey a simple yet hopeful message: "You are not alone. You matter to us. We are here for you."

References

1. Substance Abuse and Mental Health Services Administration. *SAMHSA's Concept of Trauma and Guidance for a Trauma-Informed Approach.* HHS Publication No. (SMA) 14-4884. Rockville, MD: SAMHSA; 2014.

2. Hallenbeck J, Goldstein MK, Mebane EW. Cultural considerations of death and dying in the United States. *Clin Geriatr Med.* 1996;12(2):393–406.

3. Geertz C. Religion as a cultural system. In: Banton M, ed. *Anthropological Approaches to the Study of Religion.* ASA Monographs 3. London: Tavistock Publications; 1966:1–46.

4. Tervalon M, Murray-García J. Cultural humility versus cultural competence: a critical distinction in defining physician training outcomes in multicultural education. *J Health Care Poor Underserved.* 1998;9(2):117–125.

5. Partain DK, Ingram C, Strand JJ. Providing appropriate end-of-life care to religious and ethnic minorities. *Mayo Clinic Proc.* 2017;92(1):147–152.

6. North Atlantic Treaty Organization (NATO) Joint Medical Committee. *Psychosocial Care for People Affected by Disasters and Major Incidents: A Model for*

Designing, Delivering and Managing Psychosocial Services for People Involved in Major Incidents, Conflict, Disasters and Terrorism. Brussels: NATO; 2008.

7. Sheppard B, Rubin GJ, Wardman JK, Wessely S. Terrorism and dispelling the myth of a panic prone public. *J Public Health Policy*. 2006;27(3):219–245.

8. Bonanno GA, Mancini AD. The human capacity to thrive in the face of potential trauma. *Pediatrics*. 2008;121(2):369–375.

9. World Health Organization, War Trauma Foundation, and World Vision International. *Psychological First Aid: Guide for Field Workers*. Geneva: World Health Organization; 2011.

10. Hobfoll SE, Watson P, Bell CC, et al. Five essential elements of immediate and mid-term mass trauma intervention: empirical evidence. *Psychiatry*. 2007;70(4):283–315.

11. Bermer M, Jacobs A, Layne C, et al. *Psychological First Aid Field Operations Guide*. 2nd ed. Rockville, MD: National Child Traumatic Stress Network; and White River Junction, VT: National Center for PTSD; 2006.

12. Mitchell KR, Anderson H. *All Our Losses, All Our Griefs: Resources for Pastoral Care*. Louisville, KY: Westminster John Knox Press; 1983.

13. Thieleman K. Epilogue: grief, bereavement, and ritual across cultures. In: Cacciatore J, DeFrain J, eds. *The World of Bereavement: Cultural Perspectives on Death in Families*. New York: Springer; 2015:287–298.

14. Davis EB, Kimball CN, Aten JD, et al. Faith in the wake of disaster: a longitudinal qualitative study of religious attachment following a catastrophic flood. *Psychol Trauma* [published online December 27, 2018]. doi:10.1037/tra0000425

15. Cherry KE, Sampson L, Galea S, et al. Spirituality, humor, and resilience after natural and technological disasters. *J Nurs Scholarsh*. 2018;50(5):492–501.

16. Shannonhouse LR, Bialo JA, Majuta AR, et al. Conserving resources during chronic disaster: impacts of religious and meaning-focused coping on Botswana drought survivors. *Psychol Trauma*. 2019;11(2):137–146.

17. Steinhauser KE, Fitchett G, Handzo GF, et al. State of the science of spirituality and palliative care research part I: definitions, measurement, and outcomes. *J Pain Symptom Manage*. 2017;54(3):428–440.

18. Ashley WWC Sr, Samet RL, Radillo R, Ali UNA, Billings D, Davidowitz-Farkas Z. Cultural and religious considerations. In: Ashley WWC Sr, Roberts SB, eds. *Disaster Spiritual Care: Practical Clergy Responses to Community, Regional and National Tragedy*. 2nd ed. Nashville, TN: SkyLight Paths; 2017:249–266.

19. Taylor J. Spiritual first aid. In: Ashley WWC Sr, Roberts SB, eds. *Disaster Spiritual Care: Practical Clergy Responses to Community, Regional and National Tragedy*. 2nd ed. Nashville, TN: SkyLight Paths; 2017:128–141.

Chapter 17

A Trauma-Informed Response to Working in Humanitarian Crises

Focus on Providers

Jessi Humphreys and Denah M. Joseph

Why Trauma-Informed Care?

Child soldiers forcibly separated from families, fed amphetamines and compelled to engage in violent acts. Twelve-year-olds sold into slavery or sexual trafficking. Third-degree burns covering the body of a young mother unable to nurse her child. Amputated limbs left lying in public spaces. Ground covered in bodies as far as the eye can see. Human cries of pain, with minimal pain medicine available. Refugees isolated in camps without access to food or water.

These are just a random selection of images of human beings' experiences of humanitarian crises. Our fellow human beings are going through intense suffering, and those of us working in humanitarian crises are likely not only to be moved by compassion but also to be traumatized by the exposure to such intense suffering. This is especially true in global health, where providers routinely and selflessly promote the welfare of others and, in doing do, can suffer unexpected harm.[1]

It is common and temporarily adaptive to proceed as if we are immune to this intensity of suffering and trauma, to focus on the immediate needs of the day, and to set our own well-being aside. While this may be effective and even necessary during a shift where primary attention is required for applying tourniquets and avoiding bullets, this is not sustainable practice for practitioners who wish to continue in the field of humanitarian medicine. Nowhere are healthcare providers as subject to as many varied forms of stress and trauma as in humanitarian crises.[2,3]

The practice of medicine exposes providers routinely to suffering and trauma even outside of crisis situations. In responding as we aspire to, with empathy and compassionate action, we recognize that vicarious or secondary trauma is invariable. The construct of trauma exposure syndrome provides a useful model for addressing the mental health sequelae for providers experiencing trauma both during and after their work in the field. Trauma response is increasingly recognized as a normal response to an abnormal situation. It may be less pathologized among healthcare providers, who tend not to think of themselves as suffering from a psychiatric disorder such as depression.

The special circumstances of caring for those in mass humanitarian crises must lead us to re-examine and redefine what exactly we can hope for in terms of burnout prevention and resilience promotion under these intense and extreme circumstances. Unique, non-normative experiences in humanitarian crises can lead to a variety of maladaptive behavioral responses, including complicated grief, substance abuse, risky sexual behavior, and numbing and dissociation.[4] These experiences are associated with and can lead to more complex stress response syndromes, including burnout, depression, trauma exposure syndrome, and anxiety-related syndromes.[5,6]

These syndromes have an impact on providers professional and personal lives, their ability to provide care to patients, and their ability to care for themselves, their families, and loved ones.[7] Addressing this is an ethical issue, as we have a moral obligation to ensure we are not sacrificing our own on the altar of caring for others in great need. It is also an imminently practical issue, as we have an interest in ensuring that our healthcare work force continues to function and provide quality care in humanitarian crises. The prime directive of being a first responder is not to become a victim yourself. We have the opportunity to be at the forefront of this movement, to recognize the risks to teams and individuals, and develop best practices in protecting providers.

Possible Psychological Syndromes in Healthcare Providers in Humanitarian Crises

Burnout

Burnout is characterized by three categories of loss[8]:
- Energy, leading to exhaustion and emotional and physical depletion
- Compassion, leading to apathy and cynicism
- Efficacy, leading to disengagement and ineffectiveness

A provider suffering from burnout might say, "What started out as important, meaningful and challenging work, becomes unfulfilling and meaningless."

Signs and symptoms of burnout include diminished empathy; more adverse events (mistakes or poor judgment); working less or leaving the profession altogether; heightened irritability; and social isolation or inability to speak of one's pain.

Depression

Signs and symptoms of depression include depressed mood, feelings of sadness, guilt, anhedonia, rumination; self-criticism and low self-worth; difficulty thinking; and suicidal ideation or action.

PTSD

Signs and symptoms of PTSD include persistent and frightening thoughts and memories of the experience; behavioral effects, such as substance and alcohol use, damage to personal relationships, depression, and suicide; and chronic illness.[9–11]

Grief

Signs and symptoms of grief comprise emotional intensity and lability, and waves of painful feelings followed by periods of emotional quietude. Usually self-esteem is not impaired as it is with depression. Grief is often confused with depression and may overlap with it, but not necessarily.

Anxiety Disorders

Signs and symptoms include repetitive thoughts and obsessions, distressing emotions ranging from fears to panic, and compulsive behaviors.

All the principles of psychological and spiritual first aid aimed toward caring for patients with psychosocial and spiritual suffering outlined in Chapter 16 apply equally to providers.

Unique Stressors for Healthcare Providers in Humanitarian Medicine

- **Death and loss**: Death is often framed as a failure in the healthcare field in general, and in particular in humanitarian crises. The extensive onslaught of death and loss of patients as well as possible loss of colleagues is unique in mass crises. Providers also uniquely experience "unnecessary deaths and injury": the phenomenon of watching individuals die or come to harm who might not die in an alternate location, time, or situation with a different set of resources. This may engender inner conflict and moral distress between ones' internal sense of justice and what one externally observes.

- **Personal safety and basic needs**: Accessing shelter, food, water; avoiding harm from human-made and natural violence; and avoiding infection (e.g., Ebola, infectious outbreaks, war and conflict areas, ongoing mass injury such as with flooding) are all stressors for workers in humanitarian crises.

- **Physical stress**: Sleep deprivation and exhaustion, the extent to which providers may work without sleep or breaks, may be extreme in humanitarian crises.

- **Moral distress**: Observing social disparities in access to medical resources can produce distress.

- **Sense of endlessness of work**: The inability to truly "finish" a day's work creates an internal struggle with the need to place boundaries around the work and focus on self-preservation, while also observing an endless line of patients, many of whom may die before being seen.

- **Vicarious trauma through recognizing suffering**: Providers experience total pain vicariously in observing physical, emotional, existential, and spiritual suffering.

- **Witnessing physical disfiguration and morbidity**: These include severe skin syndromes such as Stevens-Johnson syndrome, tetanus, burns, damage to and loss of limbs, facial disfiguration and loss of vision, and injuries related to weapons that have characteristic mutilating effects (e.g., from improvised explosive devices [IEDs], machetes, chemical weapons).

- **Witnessing mortality and morbidity of children**: This involves witnessing death, injury, physical disfiguration, and abandonment of children.

- **Isolation**: Providers may be isolated either from colleagues or from other providers; they are typically far away from their families, loved ones, or personal sources of support.

- **Lack of autonomy and voice for dissent**: The response to a crisis may be orchestrated by a number of organizations, with different resourcing, goals, and leadership structures. Orders may come from unclear locations, and providers may have minimal insight into or control over how and when decisions are made, often without a venue to express concerns.

- **Team-related stressors**: These include unclear roles, expectations, and leadership.

- **Existential suffering**: Observing these forms of trauma can trigger providers to question their meaning or purpose, as well as why these traumas occur.

- **Challenges in measuring and reducing suffering**: There may be a paucity of ways in which to quantify suffering, thus challenging organizations to measure and decrease this metric. Humanitarian aid organizations may measure the number of deaths, but may not measure the number of deaths with high levels of pain or suffering, challenging one's ability to improve this outcome.

Resilience in the Context of Caring for Those Affected by a Humanitarian Crisis

Humanitarian crises engender unique sources of trauma for individuals and teams providing care in these settings. Given the striking impacts of trauma, basic knowledge needs to be shared with healthcare providers in humanitarian crises situations—that trauma syndromes are both an occupational hazard and, with training and practice, a preventable or reducible harm.

Definitions of resilience for healthcare providers usually address one's ability to respond to stress in an adaptive way, the ability to "bounce back," and "the rapidity with which one recovers from adversity."[12]

One core way to think about trauma exposure in healthcare is to recognize the signs of dysregulation of one's own nervous system and to learn timely interventions aimed at this dysregulation and hyperarousal that can be used in the field to help ameliorate some of these symptoms.

The skills and practices needed for sustainable caregiving under normal circumstances may be quite different from those needed in crisis situations, where there are added barriers, including tremendous time pressures and urgency to providing care, lack of needed resources, lack of functional lines of communication, and highly stressful conditions such as chaos and danger. A provider is unlikely to be able to use most resilience tools that are gaining traction in current medical training, such as reflective practice, mindfulness, and positive psychology interventions such as gratitude and appreciation. We must tailor our approach to resiliency in the context of these limitations.

A Moment of Self-Compassion	Practicing "The Pause"
Silently say to yourself, "I am doing my very best in this difficult situation, and that is good enough. All human beings suffer. We are in this together."	Stop, take one deep breath slowly, feeling your breath in your lungs and your feet on the ground.

Grounding	Attention Management
Take a few moments to notice your physical self; scan the body slowly from head to toe for tension. Notice it without judgment. Feel your feet on the ground. Connect with the strength that comes from the earth. Then move around and break the circuit!	Shift your focus from the crisis situation to something that is not charged. Go outside for a few minutes, look out a window, close your eyes, say a prayer or blessing silently.

Figure 17.1. Resiliency practices.

Resiliency Practices in the Field for Providers

Figure 17.1 provides some examples of ways to practice resilience in the field. Other methods are as follows:

- **Brief debriefing**: Discuss events or experiences, build connections between team members, recognize each others' emotional experience; name what you are experiencing without fear of reprisal.
- **Acknowledge emotional response to an event**: Emotional processing can be done as time allows to relieve distress and emotional numbing and exhaustion. Name and acknowledge emotions being felt.
- **Short mindful practices**: These involve grounding, taking a mindful breath, practicing "the pause."[13]
- **Self-compassion**: Acknowledge your limitations in the context of mass suffering.

Practices in the Field for the Team

The most critical thing team leaders can do to support team members is to build mutual trust and psychological safety.[14] Trust and a sense of safety are the bedrock of all teams in palliative care, even more so in humanitarian crises in which providers may be activated and dysregulated emotionally much of the time. Some ways to establish trust and a sense of safety include the following:

- **Team debriefing**: Whether in the field or afterward, impromptu or planned, 5 minutes or 30, having a process that provides for the psychological safety of all participants is essential.[15] Emphasize effective, open, and respectful communication. Practice and model inclusivity and diversity of discipline. Empower all members of the team to speak, and encourage everyone to give and receive feedback freely.[16] *If there is only one practice you adopt, this should be it.*

- **Model vulnerability**: Normalize how traumatic experiences impact providers (i.e., combat the belief that providers in these settings are "tough" and not affected by suffering). Emphasize common humanity and humility: "We all make mistakes, struggle with X."
- **Affirm relationships, connection, and belonging**: Focus on what the team is doing well. Express appreciation for each other. Recognize successes by all team members. Find things to be grateful for even amidst great suffering.

Practices for the Team When out of the Humanitarian Crisis Setting

When and if the crisis passes, or the provider is no longer working in the setting of the crisis, we suggest the following resilience promotion practices:

- **Team debriefing**: This involves processing grief and trauma, focusing on the emotional dimension, possibly debriefing with colleagues, or professional therapy.
- **Integrating one's experience into one's assumptive world**: This can happen through writing, storytelling, creative expression, and sharing with compassionate colleagues—this is a reflective process that takes time. Some guiding questions for reflection include the following: What moved me about my experience? What distressed me the most about my experience? What did I learn from this experience? What would I tell someone who was thinking of doing what I just did? What meaning does it hold for me that I did this? What values of mine did I understand better as a result of this experience?
- **Embracing post-traumatic growth**: It is of utmost importance that practitioners who work in the field of humanitarian medicine receive support, to make the experience positive and meaningful in the long term. Educating providers about trauma ahead of time, as well as highlighting growth after the experience, can be life-saving. Although in this chapter we have focused on the challenges of this work, we also want to emphasize the profound meaning and value it can provide to those who choose it. The majority of people ultimately *respond to trauma with healing and growth.*

A Call to Arms for Organizations

Best practice trauma-informed care requires an organizational and systemic response to recognizing the effects of trauma and providing preventative and proactive healing and treatment for providers. A complete approach would include preparative training for providers prior to being in the field, identifying experienced trauma, and providing healing practices and *mental health referrals as appropriate*, both on site as well as after returning home. This requires a fundamental overhaul of a system that has historically not acknowledged the effects of trauma on providers. It also requires a recommitment to the well-being of practitioners providing this much-needed and precious care.[17,18]

References

1. Oakley BA, ed. *Pathological Altruism*. Oxford, New York: Oxford University Press; 2012.

2. Holloway J, Everly GS. Mental health considerations for military humanitarian aid personnel. *Int J Emerg Ment Health*. 2010;12(3):193–198.

3. Strohmeier H, Scholte WF, Ager A. Factors associated with common mental health problems of humanitarian workers in South Sudan. *PLoS ONE*. 2018;13(10):e0205333. doi:10.1371/journal.pone.0205333

4. Van der Kolk BA. *The Body Keeps the Score: Brain, Mind, and Body in the Healing of Trauma*. New York: Penguin Books; 2015.

5. Ager A, Pasha E, Yu G, Duke T, Eriksson C, Cardozo BL. Stress, mental health, and burnout in national humanitarian aid workers in Gulu, northern Uganda. *J Trauma Stress*. 2012;25(6):713–720. doi:10.1002/jts.21764

6. Strohmeier H, Scholte WF. Trauma-related mental health problems among national humanitarian staff: a systematic review of the literature. *Eur J Psychotraumatol*. 2015;6:28541. doi:10.3402/ejpt.v6.28541

7. Dewa CS, Loong D, Bonato S, Thanh NX, Jacobs P. How does burnout affect physician productivity? A systematic literature review. *BMC Health Serv Res*. 2014;14:325. doi:10.1186/1472-6963-14-325

8. Maslach C, Schaufeli WB, Leiter MP. Job burnout. *Annu Rev Psychol*. 2001;52:397–422. doi:10.1146/annurev.psych.52.1.397

9. Shanafelt TD, Bradley KA, Wipf JE, Back AL. Burnout and self-reported patient care in an internal medicine residency program. *Ann Intern Med*. 2002;136(5):358–367.

10. Oreskovich MR, Shanafelt T, Dyrbye LN, et al. The prevalence of substance use disorders in American physicians. *Am J Addict*. 2015;24(1):30–38. doi:10.1111/ajad.12173

11. Lopes Cardozo B, Gotway Crawford C, Eriksson C, et al. Psychological distress, depression, anxiety, and burnout among international humanitarian aid workers: a longitudinal study. *PLoS ONE*. 2012;7(9):e44948. doi:10.1371/journal.pone.0044948

12. Connor KM, Davidson JRT. Development of a new resilience scale: the Connor-Davidson Resilience Scale (CD-RISC). *Depress Anxiety*. 2003;18(2):76–82. doi:10.1002/da.10113

13. Chemali Z, Smati H, Johnson K, Borba CPC, Fricchione GL. Reflections from the Lebanese field: "first, heal thyself." *Confl Health*. 2018;12:8. doi:10.1186/s13031-018-0144-2

14. Smith CD, Balatbat C, Corbridge S, et al. Implementing optimal team-based care to reduce clinician burnout. *NAM Perspectives*. September 2018. doi:10.31478/201809c

15. Robbins I. The psychological impact of working in emergencies and the role of debriefing. *J Clin Nurs*. 1999;8(3):263–268.

16. Mayo AT, Woolley AW. Teamwork in health care: maximizing collective intelligence via inclusive collaboration and open communication. *AMA J Ethics*. 2016;18(9):933–940. doi:10.1001/journalofethics.2016.18.9.stas2-1609

17. Wallace JE, Lemaire JB, Ghali WA. Physician wellness: a missing quality indicator. *Lancet*. 2009;374(9702):1714–1721. doi:10.1016/S0140-6736(09)61424-0

18. Shanafelt TD, Noseworthy JH. Executive leadership and physician well-being: nine organizational strategies to promote engagement and reduce burnout. *Mayo Clin Proc*. 2017;92(1):129–146. doi:10.1016/j.mayocp.2016.10.004

Index

Tables, figures and box are indicated by *t*, *f* and *b* following the page number

For the benefit of digital users, indexed terms that span two pages (e.g., 52–53) may, on occasion, appear on only one of those pages.